# Care, Compassion and Recognition: An Ethical Discussion



Carlo Leget, Chris Gastmans, Marian Verkerk (eds.)

Peeters
2011

Cover from a painting by the German Jewish painter Felix Nussbaum (1904-1944). Site of the Museum of his work: http://www.osnabrueck.de/fnh/10508.asp. Nussbaum has - while firmly rooted in the European tradition of modern art - given the atrocities of Nazism a face. We honor his life and work by pointing at his artwork on the covers of this series *Ethics of Care*.

**Felix Nussbaum**
**A Group of Three**, 1944
Oil on canvas, 102.00 x 82.00 cm
Berlin, Deutsches Historisches Museum



ISBN 978-90-429-2459-8
D/2010/0602/120

# Ethics of Care
# Volume 1
# 2011

RECOGNITION

# 1.

# *Ethics of care, compassion and recognition*

Annelies van Heijst and Carlo Leget

## 1. Introducing the ethics of care debate

The ethics of care is a relatively new phenomenon within philosophical and theological ethics. The starting point was Carol Gilligan's *In a Different Voice* (1982): a methodological and epistemological critique of Lawrence Kohlberg's model of moral development. Her main hypothesis was that Kohlberg's model reflected androcentric biases. Methodologically, white middle-class males had functioned as the standard for a human being. Epistemologically the notions of justice, individuality, and freedom (of choice), and rational abstraction functioned as the cornerstones of the model of moral development. Gilligan noticed that the answers of many women and girls fitted into the lowest scales. Therefore she asked herself: are women morally less developed or could it be that their solutions of moral dilemmas reveal a different type of moral reasoning; i.e. do they speak in a different voice that has to be understood from a yet-to-be-developed ethical "logic"?

Gilligan concluded that it was possible to discern a different type of moral reasoning. This difference, however, was not exclusively tied to gender (although more white middle-class women than white middle-class men tended to use the care-model of moral reasoning). The main characteristics of Gilligan's proposal were, firstly, that care, instead of justice, becomes a key concept; secondly, relation and interrelatedness, instead of autonomy and individuality, are central concepts; thirdly, moral deliberation does not concentrate on general abstractions but on situations in particular; fourthly, the type of rationality is not emotionally detached but emotion-informed (i.e. reflected emotions); and fifthly, dependency and inequality are main themes.

Gilligan's study provoked an intense debate in which scholars of various disciplines participated. Therefore the ethics of care is not a school or solid faction with its own members. It is, rather, a movement of allied thinkers, who have a shared concern and who reflect on similar topics. Women and men, non-whites and whites, disabled and non-disabled, western and non-western people commented on the so-called ethics of care and developed the body of knowledge.

This body of knowledge is still growing, the debate is unfinished and does not have one, well-defined outcome. The various contributors have not come up with a set of principles, rules or doctrines that form or underpin "the" ethics of care. Rather the debate itself is known as "the ethics of care": wide-ranging and differentiated as it is. Its open end refers to an epistemological critique, and to the feminist suspicion of patriarchal keepers of truth, whose followers were not allowed to alter the slightest details. Feminist thinkers show much concern about how non-sexist, non-racist and non-elitist ways of knowing can be established. Some male thinkers who reflect on care practices—in particular professional care practice—prove to be allied thinkers.

Although in the debate there is theoretical disagreement on how "justice" and "care" relate to one another, a set of common threads can be discerned:

- Anthropologically, there is agreement about dominant ethics having pictured the human person apart from his or her connectedness with other people, neglecting the narrative dimensions of identity, and overlooking the human condition of dependency. This was pointed out by Eva Feder Kittay in *Love's Labour* (1999) and in *The Subject of Care: Feminist Perspectives on Dependency* (2002); by Hilde Lindemann Nelson in *Recognition*

*Responsibility and Rights* (2003); and by Annelies van Heijst in *Models of Charitable Care: Catholic Nuns and Children in their Care in Amsterdam, 1952-2002*, (2008, published in Dutch in 2002 as *Liefdewerk*) and in *Professional Loving Care* (to be published in 2011, published in Dutch in 2005 as *Menslievende zorg*). Flemish authors such as Axel Liégeois, Chris Gastmans, Linus Vanlaere and Mieke Grypdonck have published on the theme of health care for especially vulnerable groups such as those suffering from dementia, people with a mental disability, psychiatric patients and people who are terminally ill.

- Socio-politically, there is consensus—thanks to Joan Tronto's influential study *Moral Boundaries* (1993)—on the distribution of care arrangements as indicators for the unequal and unjust distribution of social power. People, mostly female and non-white people, who provide direct care and perform dirty and heavy care labor, have low social status and are underpaid. This analysis can be applied on a global perspective as well—as Fiona Robinson has shown in *Globalizing Care* (1999).
- Epistemologically, there is consensus that the ethics of care should relate to current mainstream ethics; see, for instance, Christa Schnabl's interpretation of Rawls and Honneth in *Gerecht Sorgen* (2005) and Margaret Walker's interpretations of Sidgwick and Strawson in *Moral Understandings* (1998).

## 2. Towards an expert seminar on care, compassion and recognition

The ethicists of care are allied thinkers who live in different countries. Three geographical areas show a slightly dissimilar development, though there are many common issues too. These three areas are The Netherlands and Belgium, Germany and Austria, and Anglo-American (and Scandinavian) regions. It is characteristic of the Dutch and Flemish ethics of care discussion that its focus is on *professional health care situations* in general (Manschot, Verkerk 1994; Verkerk 1997; Baart 2001; Grypdonck 2002; Leget 2003; Vorstenbosch 2005; Gastmans, Vanlaere 2005; Liégeois 2005). It is typical of the German and Austrian debate to concentrate on the *gendered division of care tasks in the private realm and the role of governments* in that respect (Wendel 2003; Schnabl 2005). The Anglo-American discussion covers both fields and also contains the valuable input from *disability* studies (Meyers 1997).

The ethics of care intends not to be a romantic utopian discourse set apart from socio-political reality. Care can only be revalued and take its societal place if existing asymmetrical power relations are unveiled, and if the dignity of care givers and care receivers is better guaranteed, socially, politically and personally. An unresolved issue in the ethics of care is how to interpret the asymmetry that is inherent in care-situations, on an interpersonal and on a political level. Summarized, ethicists of care, and certainly various other ethicists as well, agree on these points:

- asymmetry (socio-political and personal) is acknowledged in the situation of direct care-providers who are unpaid or underpaid, and lack social recognition;
- asymmetry (socio-political and personal) is acknowledged in the situation of care receivers who depend on other people; direct care providers may have a low position in social hierarchy but often the care receivers occupy an even less powerful position;
- the fake symmetry of the neo-liberal and economic client-model that has become current in the health care and well fare sector is exposed ;
- the actual egalitarian standard of "equality" as the equivalent of "dignity" is identified and attacked, and the problem that follows from that standard is identified: those who are evidently unequal will not count as dignified human beings.

In order to contribute to the ongoing discussion on the ethics of care, on May 24 and 25, 2007 an expert seminar was organized by the Department of Religious Studies and Theology of the University of Tilburg in collaboration with the Expert Center of Care Ethics that is located in the University Medical Center Groningen. In the preparation for this event three central issues were identified for future research. Firstly, the articulation from a care perspective of the moral dimensions of symmetry and asymmetry in the personal and socio-political domain. Secondly, the evaluation of the moral significance of the concepts of "recognition" (not yet known) and "compassion" in relation to a/symmetry within care situations. And thirdly, the reconsideration of "recognition" and "compassion" from an ethics of care perspective.

### *Recognition: "Anerkennung" as expressed in the theory of Axel Honneth*

In order to reflect on the theme of recognition, the organizing committee chose to focus on the work of the German philosopher Axel Honneth. In the last decade Axel Honneth has set out the milestones for a theory of recognition ("Anerkennung") and objectivation ("Verdinglichung") in various works (Honneth 1992/2003 and 2005). As for care situations, Honneth has contributed to the discussion by central insights such as: highlighting the relation between struggle and recognition; pointing to the elementary relevance of recognition in the sense of noticing there is some*one* there, instead of some*thing*; mapping out that recognition cannot be retrieved but results from conflicts; and (although Honneth himself does not classify this as a *care* relationship) attributing a central place to a care relationship in the theory of recognition, namely, the relation between the primary caretaker and the young child, that enables the child to become decentered, to identify with others, and observe and know the world as something apart from him.[1]

Although Honneth introduces promising insights for the ethics of care concerning a/symmetry (personal and political), there are also questions to be further reflected upon. Does Honneth's theory contribute, e.g., to the question of how care providers can gain recognition on a political and personal level? And does the theory help us to reinterpret the asymmetrical position of dependent people in moral terms?

More fundamentally, Honneth can be questioned by insights from the ethics of care. In Honneth's theory the primary caretaker-child relation is foundational, since knowing is preceded by recognition. Yet, Honneth does not describe this caretaker-child relation in terms of care, rather in terms of psychological development. (As if this were a natural fact and not the result of the care investment of the primary caretakers.) Many ethicists of care would approach this from two different angles. They would question the mother-child relationship as a foundational metaphor in ethics. And they would point to the significance of care as a practice of efforts and of responsibility, instead of something that is naturally there. Children do not love their primary caretakers out of the blue, but in response to careful treatment, which is an investment of labor, attention and relationship.

### *Compassion: "la pitié" as developed by Emmanuel Housset*

In order to reflect on the theme of compassion, the organizing committee chose to focus on the work of French philosopher Emmanuel Housset. Recently, Housset has outlined a theory of compassion—or pity, as the French word "la pitié" would probably be translated best (Housset 2003). In his phenomenological approach he states that there is always something unbearable about pity, yet a person without pity would be almost inhuman. This paradox reveals the necessity of examining the essence of pity, in order to distinguish fake pity—dangerous and disdainful—from that which comprises our humanity. Recognition of authentic pity, which respects others in their irreplaceable singularity and provides us with the intelligence of what we must do for them, allows us to free ourselves from both moralism and from an abstract rational morality, in order to envisage a tangible ethic in which the human community is, above all, one of suffering and joy.

Concerning care situations, three central insights of Housset were identified as the point of departure for further reflection. The first insight concerns the concept of compassion or pity as a pre-moral asymmetrical notion. Housset defines pity as the awareness of being touched, not as an emotion but as a bodily phenomenon. Secondly,

Housset warns of the danger of fake compassion, or pity as egoism in disguise (*malivola benevolentia*). He takes as his basis Augustine's "*malivola benevolentia*" (the happiness of do-goodism, combined with a sigh of relief that the helper or caretaker is not in that unlucky position herself). And thirdly, Housset speaks of an original "community of misery" ("communauté de la misère") and articulates a radical symmetry between human beings, rooted in an originary experience ("expérience originaire") of participating in life and being part of a common world. According to him, we are like others in the sense that we are not transparent to ourselves and are not able to direct autonomously the course of our life. If we defend this, we will open a path towards radical symmetry of ourself and the other in terms of fellowship: we are both members of the human race, humankind, or family of men.

Housset's central insights resulted in three sets of questions that were central to the preparation of the seminar: firstly, can Housset help to understand the nature of the asymmetrical dimension of what goes on between care providers and care receivers, or should we conclude that the dimension he refers to is skipped in professional care practice and in private care practice? Secondly, can Housset's theory help to unravel fake compassion in care situations? What should care providers begin to see? An thirdly, can Housset's theory help to articulate a common ground for care providers and people in their care, not founded upon a discourse of rights and justice, but upon a shared lack of transparency to oneself and our inability to be in total control of our lives?

## 3. The contributions in this volume

The lectures and discussions that were held in the expert seminar have resulted in the following series of contributions. Their common interest is that they all circle around the themes of care, compassion and recognition. They are the result of a discussion between ethicists from different cultures and continents, yet all are convinced that care is a basic human activity that continues to be worth reflecting on in order to "maintain, continue and repair our "world" so that we can live in it as well as possible" (Fisher and Tronto 1990). In order to facilitate the journey of the reader of this volume, the contributions collected here are organized in three sections: foundations, compassion and recognition.

### *Foundations*

This series of contributions opens with three articles that concern the foundation of the debate by understanding what caring means in a human life (Vanlaere, Gastmans), questioning the starting assumptions (Tronto), and critically reflecting on the narrative social activity that morality basically is (Lindemann).

Linus Vanlaere and Chris Gastmans, open the first series of contributions by focusing on the central issue of care. In their contribution they aim to enhance the understanding of what caring means in human life via a review of the philosophical-ethical literature. To do justice to the complex and multidimensional character of care, several fundamental characteristics of care are outlined, instead of providing a central definition of care. The four fundamental care features that are discussed are: firstly, care is a way of life and, at the same time, an ethical task; secondly, care is a practice that combines attitude and activity; thirdly, care is reciprocal; and fourthly, care is meaning-giving. In their analysis every step they take is field-tested by considering nursing as an example. Thus is shown that a thorough description of each one of these alone seems to require a consideration of the other three features.

Joan Tronto continues the discussion by challenging some of the preliminary assumptions contained within the framing of the issues of the seminar in terms of the possibility of *pitié*/compassion and *Anerkennung*/recognition helping to provide a basis for counterbalancing inequalities in care. She argues that one needs to be more specific about some realities of care before one can determine which philosophical conceptions might be useful. Not all care receivers are dependent, not all care providers are disregarded in society; the arrows of care dependence can point in both directions. While *pitié* and *Anerkennung* are helpful concepts to use in thinking about care, they are not, by themselves, sufficient to overcome the biases that create asymmetry in care. Furthermore, not all care is asymmetrical, and perhaps we make a mistake when we use asymmetrical care as our model. Subsequently Tronto argues and shows that unless care is placed into a democratic, political context, these or other dilemmas about caring cannot be resolved.

Hilde Lindemann, finally, broadens the scope from compassion and recognition to a fundamental reflection on the nature of morality. In order to unseat the Enlightenment model in favor of a unique narrative ethics, she focuses on examining a number of claims that have been made in the last twenty years or so concerning the moral work that narratives are capable of. To organize the claims under examination, she takes up seven sorts of things that can be done with stories. The first thing one can do with stories is read them. Second, one can invoke them. Third, one can compare them. Fourth, one can construct them. Fifth, one can counter them. Sixth, one can analyze them. And seventh, one can parody them. After she has discussed the moral purposes to which each of these narrative acts can be put, Lindemann offers her own account of the differences between Enlightenment and narrative approaches to ethics. Any judgment as to whether stories can do the various kinds of moral work that are claimed for them depends on what, precisely, one takes morality to be. In her view morality is something we do together: it is a socially embodied medium of understanding and adjustment in which people engage in practices of allotting, assuming, or deflecting responsibilities of various kinds.

### *Compassion*

After the three foundational contributions, four subsequent articles focus on the theme of compassion. Emanuel Housset opens the debate with an article on the paradoxes of pity, which can be read as a shorter version of the French monograph he published in 2005. Housset begins by sketching the paradox of pity: it is at the same time insufferable and indispensable, dangerous and a deliverance. It is exactly this paradoxical nature which makes it a privileged entry point for a phenomenological analysis in three steps. In a first step Housset pleads for the necessity of a concrete ethics. He rejects overhasty classifications and discovers pity to be a phenomenon anterior to intersubjectivity. In a second step, Housset makes efforts to analyze what he calls "dangerous pity." Drawing on Nietzsche's refusal of pity, he distinguishes between good pity and bad pity. This opens the way to a re-evaluation of pity, the understanding of human weakness included. By means of conclusion he states that the decisive paradox of pity is that it is a sentiment that does not lock us up in ourselves but that, on the contrary, leads us to exist beyond ourselves by widening our sensitivity to that distance (*lointain*) that is the other, and this prior to any decision.

Mieke Grypdonck, in her contribution, examines recognition and pity in relation to nursing care for persons suffering from a chronic disease, in particular for the field of what has come to be called self-management. Where in medical circles self-management is often considered (from the perspective of care givers and health policy) to be synonymous with adherence, Grypdonck adopts the patient's perspective and shows that it is a hard and demanding practice. Making efforts to really understand what moves people to be non-adherent, e.g. to fluid restriction, asks for recognition in the full sense. It asks for real interest in how people's lives are organized and in the story that lies behind their lives. After having elaborated on the importance of recognition, Grypdonck takes up the subject of pity. Although she understands that there are good reasons why pity is not a popular concept, not in the least because of the asymmetry associated with it, Grypdonck follows Housset in distinguishing between bad and good pity. The latter, as a virtue, is positive only if moderated by sensitivity and thoughtfulness.

Carlo Leget also builds on the analysis of Housset, applying the latter's ideas to the context of education in an academic medical centre and moves in two directions. First he thinks along with Housset. As an introduction into the world of medicine he gives an impression of the problems one meets teaching ethics to medical students and explains why he thinks Housset's analysis is worth taking to heart. In short, Housset's view on compassion helps in formulating an answer to four widespread ideas that hamper ethical conversations before they have really begun: emotivism, legalism, consequentialism, and misplaced tolerance. Secondly, taking the other direction, he proposes four critical questions that help in performing a further analysis in order to determine the right place of compassion in an ethics of care. These questions concern: firstly, the power and impact of the health care system; secondly, the problem of justice; thirdly, the place of negative emotions; and fourthly, the question whether compassion is really needed and it is better to confine oneself to the concept of empathy.

Axel Liégeois addresses the research question whether one can use the concept of compassion to deal with the asymmetry in the care-relationship. He gives a response from the specific perspective of professional care for people with intellectual disability, developing the following reflection. Firstly, he presents the two assumptions of the research question, namely the asymmetry in the care relationship and the concept of compassion. Then he draws the perspective of intellectual disability care in which the citizenship-paradigm with the key concept of empowerment is actually prominent. From this perspective he develops a critical reflection and a short inquiry among professional care providers on the concept of compassion. Consequently, Liégeois argues in favour of an integrative approach of compassion and empowerment in care ethics. He suggests that the new concept of "empowering compassion" would help to handle the asymmetry in the care-relationship. Empowering compassion is the respectful awareness of being touched by the other's suffering and the growing empowerment to alleviate this suffering.

### *Recognition*

The last section of this book is dedicated to the exploration of the subject of recognition in relation to care ethics. Christa Schnabl elaborates the socio-political organization of care in a just and righteous way with regard to gender, class and ethnicity. Women and immigrants are the social groups that have been burdened with care work, which was often unpaid, underpaid or not rewarded, Schnabl's main question is whether and how the ethics of care can help to improve the value of care and modify care relations so that they turn into just relations. She values Honneth's theory of recognition as an enlargement of modernity's ethical universalism but thinks he is not radical enough. She argues that Honneth's view leads to ethical dualism, in which justice and care each represent an ethical logic of their own resulting in a justice-care antagonism. In trying to overcome this opposition Schnabl offers a view of *justified care* in which care receiving is defined in a facetted way. It is an obligation among family members which should be realized in a just way; it is a social virtue in the context of neighborhood and civil society; and it is a human right for all people who need support. The three aspects mentioned concern those who need care. However, care givers are also integrated in Schnabl's ideal of justified care as they should be protected against exclusion, exploitation and discrimination.

Estelle Ferrarese searches for the shared premisses of the ethics of care and theories of recognition, which she locates in the moral category of "vulnerability". Ferrarese places Honneth in the theoretical surrounding of the Frankfurt Schule, of which he is a current representative. Ferrarese does so, by presenting several of these thinkers and their shared concern for a body of theory that is sensitive to the "microcosmology", i.e. situations in their particularity and non-universalistic way of being. Reconstructing Honneth's view on care, Ferrarese concludes that his theory of recognition and the ethics of care are to a certain extent incompatible grammars. Nevertheless, she detects a shared common denominator which lies in the concept of vulnerability. She finds such an overlap in the underlying anthropology of vulnerability in both theories of recognition and the ethics of care. Care ethics have illuminated the importance of the difference between potential and materialized vulnerabilities. The latter type of vulnerability calls for more than a negative answer, namely care in the full sense of the word. Nonetheless, theories of recognition invite us to broaden the concept of justice, because not only the right of physical integrity is acknowledged but also the right of satisfying conditions for a positive relationship to self. Social and moral theories should take into consideration that moral and mental wounds are likely to be inflicted and this calls for political and social transformations.

Margaret Urban Walker focuses on the concept of recognition through the lens of a reflection on human dignity. Dignity, she argues, is a moral ideal that by tradition belongs to a tight circle of concepts including rational agency, autonomous choice, humanity, respect, rights, recognition, and moral worth. Influenced heavily by the Kantian legacy, contemporary thinking often identifies dignity with full or fully mature capacities for moral agency. Walker examines the idealized and exclusive results of so viewing dignity, and suggests three strategies: naturalizing dignity, rendering dignity relationally, and differentiating the responses that affirm dignity. These strategies can render the moral ideal of dignity more inclusive and humane, while preserving the importance of normal human capacities for mutual accountability.

Andries Baart and Frans Vosman complete this section on recognition with a series of two articles that focus on relation-based care and recognition. Both articles are written as a contribution to the discussion on the quality of care, a search for quality that has become a search for technical provisions. In this discussion, practical and fundamental moral aspects of quality of care have been obscured, to the detriment of the concept of quality of care itself.

In the first article, "Sketching good care from the theory of presence and five entries" a theoretical framework developed by Andries Baart is introduced, *i.e.* the theory of presence. Baart's presence theory is sketched as encompassing a professional way of doing (methodology), a cultural critique, an explicit normative perspective on care, a paradigmatic shift in producing relevant and sound knowledge about care giving, and a characteristic interpretation of societal injustice and human suffering (and human dignity). The presence theory is considered much more than a new alternative method. It may be interpreted as the (nowadays frequently forgotten and pushed aside) basis of all interventionist intentions—its critical memory, its ultimate legitimacy and its proper frame of relevance (what it is all about). In a second step, Baart and Vosman give attention to five (types of) "entries" to the quality of care debate: objective needs, foundation standards, consumer experiences, radically patient centred approaches and a last entry that comprises a political critical perspective and leads to the second article.

In the second article, "Good care and recognition" Vosman and Baart further elaborate on the question "what makes care good care?" according to the theory of presence. The authors distinguish six characteristics that also form the backbone of their contribution. Good care must have the proper identity, that is, it must actually *be* care; it must be relevant, that is, fine-tuned to the specified needs; it must be true, that is, effective; it must be legitimate in more respects than just legal; it must be doable, technically and humanly speaking; and good care is beneficence, a caring good in itself and *sui generis*. After having outlined their idea of good care, in six paragraphs they elucidate and analyze these characteristics. With the contributions of Baart and Vosman we are back at the starting point of our tour: a view on what makes care good care.

## Notes

[1] Honneth refers in this respect to the work of Piaget, Mead, Cavell and Tomasello (Honneth 2005, 46-61).

# 2.

# *To be is to care: a philosophical-ethical analysis of care with a view from nursing*

Linus Vanlaere and Chris Gastmans

In the last few decades, care has played an increasingly crucial role in human self-understanding. Consideration of the concept of care has given rise to increased attention on its meaning in ethical theory (Little 1998), resulting in the formal development of care ethics, an ethical perspective that considers care to be an ethical value. Since being developed in moral psychology (Gilligan 1982) and political theory (Tronto 1993), care ethics has been immensely influential in health care (Jecker & Reich 2004). In nursing, for example, care ethics is used to make the intrinsic ethical meaning of daily care processes more explicit (Davis & Fowler 2006; Gastmans et al. 1998).

Care as a key concept in care ethics, however, has faced much criticism (Allmark 1995; Crigger 1997; Gaul 1995; Nelson 1992; Paley 2002). A major critique is that the meaning of care remains unclear. If a specific domain is not first delimited—for example, the domain of nursing—the notion of care can be a very vague concept. To ensure that the concept of care can function meaningfully in ethical discourse, we need to exert intellectual effort in defining it.

In this chapter, we try to enhance our understanding of what caring in human life means through a thorough review of the philosophical-ethical literature. We field-test the meaning of care by considering nursing as an example. Since care is a complex phenomenon from which we do not want to strip its versatility, we found it useful to formulate several essential care features that describe the concept rather than to create a universal definition of care. The four fundamental care features that we consider are: (1) care is simultaneously a way of life and an ethical task; (2) care is a practice that combines attitude and activity; (3) care is reciprocal; and (4) care is meaning-giving. These four fundamental features are interwoven, from which emerges an overarching synthesis of the concept of care. Although these features cannot be separated if we are to maintain a complete understanding of care, we nonetheless must delineate and discuss them in succession for clarification.

## 1. Care is a fundamental way of life and an ethical task

The concept of care refers to a certain value in human life. Care concerns the way people cope with vulnerabilities intrinsic to life and the way they handle the reciprocal dependence that these vulnerabilities entail. Care as a value normally refers to a positive qualification: attentiveness to the needs and wants of another. However, in human life, care first appears as a way of life and not as an ethical task. How should we interpret these two aspects—way of life vs. ethical task—of care?

### *Care as a fundamental way of life*

In its broadest sense, care can be defined as a fundamental way of life.[1] In the domain of human activity, care as a fundamental way of life includes all facilitating gestures made by people to improve the human condition or way of life. It represents everything a person does to live a life fitting of humanity. Care is one of the most important manifestations of daily life: by means of numerous care activities, people can endure in life (Van Hooft 1995; Nussbaum 2002). This sense of the concept of care can also be found in the definition of Joan Tronto (1993, 162). She develops the notion of care as an activity that includes everything that people do to ensure that their world continues to exist and can be repaired and maintained, so that it becomes "their" world where they can live in the best possible way.

According to this broad definition, care has a biological grounding. Care, in a sense, can manifest itself as an instinctive act (Van

Hooft 1995; Verhoeven 2002), one clearly observed in animals. Consider the effort a bird puts forth to feed its helpless young, a clear indication of the instinctive nature of caring. Care also emerges in its most elementary form in people as all instinctive acts in response to biological needs. However, most biologically embedded care activities of humans rarely occur spontaneously; rather, these activities are created in a human environment, an environment from which these activities take on meaning. In this way, care activities become part of being human. Indeed, according to Cornelis Verhoeven, care is "more elementary" as a fundamental way of life than as an ethical task because of its biological grounding (Verhoeven 2002, 12). Since care as a fundamental way of life can also be found in the gray area of elementary vital pleasures, pleasure is also involved in care.

A number of sociobiologists have advanced the notion that care has a biological grounding and that an "instinctive drive" exists in humans that lead to care acts (De Waal 2001, 2006; Krebs & Janicki 2004). Modern sociobiology posits that people—due to evolutionary pressures—are not egocentric by nature but are really altruistic, embracing moral standards that advance the survival of the human species. This implies that certain moral standards do not originate from one's upbringing but have biological grounding (Vine 1992). Thus, in its broadest sense, care can be considered to be a moral standard. Why? Because the tendency to care is embedded in the biological nature of humankind (Krebs & Janicki 2004). However, this does not mean that care in humans is congenital. Rather, we can say that evolution provided humankind with the *ability* to care; *whether and how* this ability develops largely depends on the surroundings in which people live and grow. After all, care takes shape through upbringing and development (De Waal 2001).

### *Care as an ethical task*

A striking element in the sociobiological discourse about care as a moral standard is that care is something worth striving toward. Here, we have a shift in meaning: if care is viewed as a moral standard, then care is no longer something that people do "by nature" or by instinct to endure in life—rather, care is an ethical task.[2] It is easy to encounter care as an ethical task in human life. When people care for and take responsibility for others, they give meaning to their life and to that of others (May 1969; Mayeroff 1971; Van Hooft 1995; Frankfurt 2004). Care is a task that adults assign to themselves; it is a task that they consider indispensable in a fulfilling life (Erikson 1964).[3] Care as an ethical task can never quite be seen as a burden imposed from the outside, but rather it is seen as a call coming from inside.

In this way, care as an ethical task rises above the "instinctive aspect" of care.[4] While care as a fundamental way of life is restricted to one's own survival and to that of one's family, care as an ethical task can also represent the care we show for people who are not directly related. With care as an ethical task, people voice an ethical commitment: they commit themselves to paying attention to and getting actively involved in the needs of others (Verhoeven 2002; Van Hooft 1995).

Although care as a fundamental way of life should be clearly distinguished from care as an ethical task, these two features of care are also linked. This link has already been demonstrated clearly in sociobiological considerations. The question is: how should we interpret this link? When the link is interpreted too narrowly, we must deal with the "naturalistic fallacy," in which "is" turns quickly into "ought" (De Waal 2001). Yet, when care as an ethical task is disconnected from care as a fundamental way of life, the danger exists that care takes on a sense of "ethical authority." In this case, one soon feels that care is a heavy burden, or even a "sacrifice." Care becomes obligatory, something that entails only effort and sacrifice, something that (certain) people *have* to do (Verhoeven 2002). Such a moralizing approach is avoided when care as an ethical task remains linked to care as a fundamental way of life, something that people do "by nature" to endure life. Since care is also a fundamental way of life, one having biological basis, care gives people elementary pleasure. Care gives pleasure because our natural need to care is linked to satisfying this need.

### *View from nursing*

The nursing literature makes a distinction between definitions that characterize care broadly as a human trait and definitions that characterize care as a moral imperative (McCance et al. 1997; Morse et al. 1990; Morse et al. 1991). Again, it boils down to the difference between care as a fundamental way of life and care as an ethical task. Definitions that view care as a human trait are often based on Heidegger's ideas (Griffin 1983; Boykin & Schoenhofer 1993; Roach 1993). Authors who define care as a moral imperative are more likely to consider care to be a moral practice (Bishop & Scudder 1990; Gastmans et al. 1998) or to be an ethical commitment (Watson 1985; Gadow 1985).

Care as a fundamental way of life normally manifests itself in everyday situations, such as self-care: it includes everything that people do to endure life. Self-care is compromised when people turn to health care. In this respect, George Agich (2003) refers to the alienating and depersonalizing influence of illness. The situation of chronically ill patients—confined to their sickbed and losing all contact with their surroundings and with their own body—is a typical example. These persons depend on others for everyday hygiene and feeding. "Strangers" take over the most intimate care acts. These persons no longer feel that they "are" somebody but rather that they have a body. They become mentally disconnected such that they view the body as a separate, unrelated object. Confronted with the loss of functional possibilities, chronically ill people are often no longer capable of leading a life in which they do things they consider valuable and or can relate to.

Starting from the definition of care as a fundamental way of life—i.e., as a tool people use to endure in life—nursing creates the necessary conditions so that an ill person can be "somebody," enabling the patient to be a person in spite of all the depersonalizing influences of being ill. To make this possible, nurses must especially consider elements that support the patient's sense of self or identity. By focusing on certain facilities, nurses can increase the patient's comfort and can ensure that the patient's functional inabilities are more or less taken care of, allowing the patient to adapt in the best possible way to the situation.

Care is not only a fundamental way of life but also a constant ethical task. It is typical for humans to respond to a call for help. For example, the goal of nursing can be described as the promotion of patient well-being by providing good care in the broader meaning of the word—i.e., on a physical level as well as psychological, relational, social, moral, and spiritual levels (Gastmans et al. 1998). This goal expresses the moral identity of nursing practice. In each situation, nurses search for appropriate ways to achieve as much good as possible for a patient or a group of patients. In every care situation, nurses have to make personal choices based on the good that nursing practice sets as a goal (Bishop and Scudder 1990).

The fact that nursing should always be grafted onto care as an ethical task means that one should also take into account the social framework in which this care develops. Caring for individuals in an immediate care relationship and caring for absent individuals—"absent third parties"—are two dimensions of the same task (Ricoeur 1990). Responding to the needs of the former individuals does not relieve nurses of responding to the needs of the latter individuals. Therefore, we should not draw a boundary between the political care policy and actual care relationships (Tronto 1993). By using political structures, we can create a health care policy that supports nurses in their ethical task of caring for "absent individuals." The care policy should be interpreted in a way that enables a balanced and fair distribution of care. This social-political mediation of care should also lead to the necessary legal and organizational facilities so that nurses could carry out their ethical care task in the best possible way (Fingeld-Connett 2007).

## 2. Care is a practice by which attitude and activity go hand-in-hand

Care can be thought of in two ways in practice: as attitudes, on the one hand, and as care activities, on the other.

### *Care: attitude and activity*

When defining care, the academic literature often distinguishes between care as an *attitude* (*caring about*) and care as an *activity* (*caring for* or *taking care of*) (Boleyn-Fitzgerald 2003; Davis & Fowler 2006; Glenn 2000; Jecker & Self 1991; Leira 1994; Silk 1998). According to the latter, care represents the activity of one person that meets the needs of another person and involves *face-to-face* interactions between both persons as crucial elements (Bubeck 1995). According to this meaning, care relates to a whole range of activities tailored to someone's well-being that also meets that person's needs.

Care as an attitude (*caring about*) refers to the mentality, feeling, and/or awareness of the care provider. It includes attention to the needs of another person (attentiveness), as well as the urge to satisfy those needs (responsibility). A person perceives that, in a given situation, something should be done for the well-being of another person. Thus, care as an attitude involves being affectionately and emotionally touched by someone in need as well as understanding (cognitive) that something should be done to address that need (Gastmans et al. 1998; Blum 1980). Care as an attitude can therefore be described as "being attentively involved" and "being devoted."

Some authors emphasize that care is an activity as well as an attitude; both aspects of care can be distinguished from one another, but they certainly cannot be separated (Davis & Fowler 2006; Jecker & Self 1991; Waerness 1987). If care is seen only as an activity, there is a real danger that an activity may be defined as caring, while attentiveness—an attitude of care provider involvement in another person's situation—will be rejected as being part of caring. Nevertheless, care is an emotional and a more comprehensive mental relationship as well, besides the purely intentional one that is expected in acts (Vorstenbosch 2005). That is why some claim that care, when defined as a set of activities, does not capture the true essence of care (Sabatino 1999). However, when care is seen only as an attitude, care can involve one's concern about the situation of another person without involving activities that express concern and actually improve the other person's situation.

When both aspects of care are combined, care is considered to be a "practice" by which activity (*caring for*) and attitude (*caring about*) go hand-in-hand. Care as a practice was first defined by Fisher and Tronto (1990, 40). According to these authors, caring is a species activity that expresses itself in specific ways of conduct—acts and attitudes—that aim to maintain, continue, and repair "our world" so that we can live in it as best as possible. In this view of care, Fisher and Tronto delineated four dimensions that can be thought of as a process with four phases. The first phase is "caring about someone or something," that is, "being worried about," "being concerned about," "paying attention to" someone or something. The care provider sees and acknowledges the care needs of the care recipient. This first step of care, of course, is linked to the ethical attitude of "attentive involvement." In the second phase, the care provider carries out real initiatives to meet the observed needs. This is the "taking care of" phase, which requires that the care provider takes responsibility for initiating care activities. Therefore, "responsibility" is the ethical attitude that corresponds with this dimension. In the third phase, the actual care giving is performed. Here, the ethical attitude of competency plays an important role. In the fourth phase, the care provider verifies whether the needs of the care recipient are effectively met. Fisher and Tronto call this the phase of "care-receiving." Paying attention to the reactions of care recipients—which is expressed in the ethical attitude of receptivity—is important to maintain quality in the care process and to motivate care providers.

This view on care corresponds in at least two ways to the characteristics of care mentioned above. First of all, the perspective of Fisher and Tronto integrates care as a fundamental way of life and as an ethical task. Care not only manifests itself as a "species activity," that is, a fundamental way of enduring in life, but also as an ethically relevant concept. Fisher and Tronto link every dimension of care to an ethical attitude. Secondly, their four dimensions of care illustrate that not only perceivable care activities but also caring attitudes are part of a complete view of care. Care acts are done on the basis of a specific ethical attitude. Attention, responsibility, competency, and receptivity are four essential attitudes acquired by people involved in care processes, if the goal is to have a complete care process.

### *View from nursing*

Some authors consider nursing, in essence, to be a practice centered on nurses' commitment to a care recipient (Austin et al. 2003; Gastmans et al. 1998). Nursing entails a number of acts based on the attempt of the nurse to understand the care recipient's situation, views, and vulnerabilities, and to handle the care recipient in the right way (McCance et al. 1997). To be able to provide good care, nurses put themselves in the care recipient's position and commit themselves to meet this situation. Nurses train to become involved with individuals they take care of. "Becoming involved with" requires nurses to be receptive toward other individuals, which means that they are really "there" for these individuals (Fingeld-Connett 2007; Austin et al. 2003).

According to Paul Van Tongeren (1999), the attitude of attentive involvement expected from nurses is "passivity" in care giving. However, "being passive" does not mean "doing nothing," as if to be likened to indolence or idleness. On the contrary, passivity in nursing means being attentive to another individual, being alert to the meaning of what happens to that individual and to what that individual's situation informs them. Care is more than just a service. It also involves "being there" when the other person needs it and in a way he/she needs it.

A nurse can acquire a caring attitude by acting in a caring way. Care practices voice an attitude of attentive involvement while developing this attitude at the same time. The fact that an attitude develops and continues to grow as one practices the *habit* of doing it, however, does not mean that caring acts are seen as *routine*. Care manifests itself exactly where tasks are done that have not been set beforehand (Fingeld-Connett 2007).

Consider, for example, two nurses: one nurse performs care acts in a professional but routine way, whereas another nurse performs care acts in a professional but less routine-like way and gives more attention to a specific situation. An uninvolved observer would probably view the second nurse to be more "caring" than the first one. The second nurse is conscientious enough to look beyond the routine tasks and to actively intervene when necessary.[5] Thus, a nurse is considered to be caring when he/she does not just carry out a standard guideline of tasks but when he/she goes beyond the standard. It is not quite possible to make up a set of criteria that care should meet, since good care typically requires that it goes beyond certain criteria.[6] Indeed, the attitude that underlies care acts is not always clear. A caring attitude results in acting when necessary. A caring nurse is capable of reacting appropriately to unexpected events.

## 3. Care is reciprocal

From our discussion of care thus far, we gather that care must be set in a relational context: people relate to each other in care relationships. In the following paragraphs, we show that the care relationship is asymmetrical as well as reciprocal.

### *Care is asymmetrical-reciprocal*

Human life is essentially relational: "Being a person" means "being connected to others" (Buber 1923). While developing into a person, we receive from others and give to others at the same time. Care, when viewed as a way in which people relate to each other, is the dialectic of giving and taking. Care consists of the needs and wants of one person and the responsibility that another person assumes to meet these needs.[7] Care always involves asymmetry: the care recipient depends on the care provider for meeting his/her specific needs. From a practical viewpoint, and sometimes from a mental and cognitive viewpoint, equality does not exist in the care relationship (Vorstenbosch 2005).

However, the care recipient is not just passive. In care relationships, care recipients always relate to care providers as their *alter ego*, that is, as a self that thinks, feels, and is free like we are free. Since care recipients are not just mere objects but subjects, in care, care recipients must be treated as persons who are capable of doing something in the world, of acting in a goal-oriented way, of sorting out priorities, and of determining goals toward which they aim their actions (Ricoeur 1990).[8] Furthermore, in care, care recipients are subjects that voice that they are subjects in the way they receive care. Here, the reciprocity of care gets its full meaning: the care recipient reciprocally gives to the care provider through the way he/she receives care.[9]

Receiving care gives rise to giving. It is exactly this giving that enriches and even completes the care provision. Therefore, receiving care is equivalent to providing care. Without recipients who respond to the care provided, care would not exist. If care recipients do not receive care and expertise from care providers, if they do not respond to it, or if they do not participate in it, then care cannot be provided (Lindemann 2003). Care only exists when it is properly provided and properly received. Thus, according to Lindemann, reciprocity is an essential part of care. If one regards care providing only as ethically relevant, then the responsibility of care receiving is denied, and therefore, the moral identity of the care recipient is also denied. For this reason Fisher and Tronto (1990) consider "care receiving" to be their fourth dimension in the care process.

### *View from nursing*

When applied to nursing, the reciprocity of care has real implications for nurses as well as for care recipients. For nurses, reciprocity should be viewed as the "communicative action" toward care recipients. Communicative action represents mainly the vehicle—speech, language, word expressions—through which reciprocity shapes a care relationship, boosting the self-respect and responsibility of care recipients (Fingeld-Connett 2007; Fredriksson & Eriksson 2003).

Initially, nurses should adopt the attitude of "moral modesty" (Smeyers 1999). Moral modesty implies that a nurse does not think that he/she can look at the care situation from the care recipient's point of view and know what the recipient needs without having to listen to the recipient. Thus, nurses cultivate an open-minded attitude toward care recipients' points of view. According to Iris Young (1997), this requires respectful "amazement": an attitude of openness vis-à-vis other people; that is, a willingness to understand the needs, interests, and values of these people.

Reciprocity also implies that care recipients have a responsibility vis-à-vis their nurses. After all, care implies that the provider, as well as the recipient, feels respected as a person. Good care can be viewed as a process by which all those concerned grow in their "person being." According to Agich (2003), care recipients show respect to their nurses by allowing themselves to be cared for and by responding appropriately to the care; for example, by expressing gratitude or by expressing displeasure. Of course, how much a care recipient assumes responsibility in the care process depends on the abilities of the recipient and on the situation (Fingeld-Connett 2007). However, Agich (2003) is convinced that respecting care recipients as moral subjects always implies their co-responsibility.

Care recipients should be aware that they exercise certain authority over care providers: they have to consider that the way they receive care has power; thus, they have to determine which attitude corresponds best to specific care situations (Lindemann 2003). In certain cases, the most appropriate ethical response is gratitude. By expressing gratitude, care recipients can direct the care process toward a very specific direction. For example, a grateful care recipient can cause a nurse to see the care situation in a more meaningful way. The result: the nurse becomes more devoted to the care provision.

Sometimes "resistant reception" can also be a proper and just ethical response. Lindemann (2003) refers to the care for adults who only get children's material in order to help them to renew certain abilities; these people can oppose this. "Resistant reception" can be a way to receive proper rehabilitative care (Lindemann 2003). When verbal defense gives little comfort and when a care recipient experiences disrespectful treatment, according to Lindemann, he/she has the moral right to resist care. The examples of gratitude and resistant reception as possible ethical responses of care recipients to care provided do not only show that care recipients have a stronger influence from an ethical point of view than what is generally assumed, but also that they have co-responsibility in care.

## 4. Care is meaning-giving

The last fundamental feature of care in our analysis is the meaning-giving aspect. Meaning is closely related to the reciprocity of care.

### *Meaning and care*

Care always relates to the dialectic between giving and taking. As Ricoeur (1990) states, the care recipient gives in a different way from the care provider: giving is not derived from the care recipient's ability to act—since he/she receives care because he/she lacks a certain ability to act—but giving is intrinsic to being open to receiving. Ricoeur considers this kind of reciprocity, in which an inequality in ability is compensated for, to be authentic reciprocity. This is the criterion par excellence of care. Depending on their own involvement and depending on the way that care recipients respond to the care provided, care providers can experience meaning (Lindemann 2003). The "asymmetry" in care is turned around: the care provider depends on the care recipient, because he/she finds certain fulfillment and meaning in the care provided. When it comes to the meaning aspect, i.e., the satisfaction to be experienced, the care provider is actually the "dependent party" in the care relationship, however paradoxical it may sound. Here, we find the true nature of human interdependence.

The meaning-giving aspect of care probably relates to "self-transcendence" in and by care, that is, a person's ability to reach out to and to connect oneself to others through care. With care as a sign of human involvement, a person's natural need to be taken away from one's center seems to be met. For it is only by acting on the behalf of others that people fully "realize" their "strengths." To find themselves, people have to go beyond themselves (Frankfurt 2004; Van Hooft 1995; Mayeroff 1971). The thing that gives life meaning is often connected to something that transcends the individual. A typical feature of self-transcendence is that the question for the proper self has become completely irrelevant and the "self" is pushed into the background, because another person is important. When transcending oneself a person becomes a bit more of himself. This paradoxical fact also embodies the meaning-giving aspect of care. Through care as an act of self-transcendence, we reach out to other people. The other person appeals to us to "do our utmost." This implies that the other person does not only offer us the possibility to "realize" what "kind of strength" we have, but that this person also offers us—without really being aware and without doing so purposely—the possibility to go beyond ourselves to be able to return to ourselves in an "enriched" way. As a consequence, the other person plays an exceptionally crucial role in our life fulfillment.

### *View from nursing*

Nursing entails involvement, contact, and interaction. This interaction can, depending on the care recipient, develop into a reciprocal care relationship. This reciprocity makes nurses feel acknowledged, not only in what they are doing but also in who they are (Fingeld-Connett 2007; Watson 2003). The reciprocity of the care relationship offers them acknowledgement of their "being a person," and that gives meaning. This is probably why nursing remains "feasible" for them. This meaning-motivation should be part of a balanced nursing option. By finding the meaning of one's life in the care of another, nurses will be able to find new strength and creativity to provide good care.

By considering the care of elderly people with dementia, Cees Hertogh (2004) showed that this satisfaction or meaningful experience is very important to nurses. Demented elderly people are prime examples of care recipients who are incapable of responding to care provided in a common way. As dementia advances, each form of personal contact that is created is torn down. A demented person's forgetfulness impedes intimacy, an intimacy that normally enables the relationship between the care recipient and nurse to grow. Hertogh notes that the patient who was most grateful in the evening for your help, will forget you in the morning and will flatly throw you out if you try to help him. However, even when caring for demented persons, nurses still stick to reciprocity in everyday contact, even if this is only an illusion. Hertogh views this as an imperative illusion, because without it caring becomes difficult since helplessness, meaninglessness, and discouragement can occur.

Although reciprocity as an ethical value in care is stressful, reciprocity remains imperative so that nurses can experience meaning in care. In practice, the stressful conditions under which nurses often have to work reduce their personal contact with care recipients. This often makes nurses feel "meaninglessness," constantly failing to meet their ideals and realize their abilities (Glasberg et al. 2007; Nordam et al. 2005). They never or hardly ever talk about their experiences and about the meaning-giving aspect that they experience in care. They work fervently to accomplish the care provision. These practices cause nurses to lose the connection between personal meaning-giving and what is asked of them.

Offering nurses tools to help them reflect on their care practice helps them to experience meaning (Hoover 2002). Becoming aware of how the care process functions teaches nurses that experiencing meaning is related to creating a story about the care recipient and that meaning-giving takes shape in a relational narrative (Rashotte 2005). By integrating the care process in a shared story, nurses can keep care from becoming meaningless.

## 5. Conclusion

Our analysis shows that care is a multiform concept. To do justice to the complex and multidimensional character of care, we have presented an outline of several fundamental characteristics of care instead of presenting a central definition. Such a definition—if it could be developed—would oversimplify the phenomenon of care. For example, care as a fundamental way of life differs in meaning from care as an ethical task. Care is a practice—activity and attitude—in which we become involved as human beings and that we use to endure in life. Furthermore, we make our life meaningful by being involved in care relationships. This meaning-giving aspect of care is linked to the reciprocity of care: the care recipient depends on the care provider to receive care and the care provider partly depends on the care recipient to experience meaning.

Care is not just the sum of its various aspects. We have to realize that an intrinsic description of care in terms of its aspects cannot be achieved by just listing a number of isolated qualities. The various components of care cannot be considered separately; they influence and evoke each other. Our analysis shows that each dimension of care seems to require each other. Thus, care can be considered to be the sum of these features, provided that we realize something essential has been added to this sum, since the sum also describes the relationships and the dynamics between the parts.

## Notes

[1] Warren Reich (2000, 2004) showed that the fundamental-way-of-life dimension of care has been already described in the Greek-Roman "*cura*-fabel," in Goethe's *Faust*, and in the works of Kierkegaard and Heidegger.

[2] Reich (2004) refers to the work of May (1969), Erikson (1964), and Mayeroff (1971) to illustrate the meaning of care as an ethical task. We also add the work of Van Hooft (1995) and Frankfurt (2004) to this list.

[3] Erik Erikson (1964) denoted care as a moral value that is crucial in human life: "Ethical adults involve themselves actively in the work of their world. Such adults maintain the world positively, holding it in trust for future generations, caring deeply and responsibly for children, for their own in an engaged, nurturing way, and for all others by their civic actions" (Hoare 2002, 72).

[4] With regards to care as an ethical task, Verhoeven stated: "Here the 'natural' altruism changes into an ethical performance which is taken on as a duty and which is considered to be a merit. There where we see the natural altruism on the borderline of its possibilities in the animal world change into a total lack of interest and where the hopeless case is mercilessly and without regret pushed aside, ethical care is given its real importance" (Verhoeven 2002, 15).

[5] The concept of "*skilled companionship*," refers to something that becomes a true success in nursing and that, as a metaphor of good nursing, aims at the indispensable integration of expertise and thoughtfulness (Titchen 2000). When a nursing task is viewed as "*skilled companionship*," professional expertise—knowledge and skills—is emphasized to be a condition for nursing. However, this expertise can lead only to good care when it is based on a caring *attitude*. The nurse's concern for the patient and his well-being is indispensable for care giving. This concern, however, should be funneled into effective care through knowledge and skills. To provide good care,

nurses should convert their professional expertise via an individual relationship into a personal answer to the patient's care question.

[6] This does not mean that care falls under the concept of "*supererogation*." It does mean, however, that good care has to do with the right reaction to the needs and wants of another person in unexpected and special circumstances. This way, care can never completely be restrained by pre-concluded criteria (Blum 1980).

[7] As Paul Ricoeur says (1990, 223): "Ici, l'initiative, en termes précisément de pouvoir-faire, semble revenir exclusivement au soi qui *donne* sa sympathie, sa compassion, ces termes étant pris au sens fort du souhait de partager la peine d'autrui. Confronté à cette bienfaisance, voire à cette bienveillance, l'autre paraît réduit à la condition de seulement *recevoir*."

[8] As Ricoeur says (1990, 226): "La similitude est le fruit de l'échange entre estime de soi et sollicitude pour autrui. Cet échange autorise à dire que je ne puis m'estimer moi-même sans estimer autrui *comme* moi-même. Comme moi-même signifie: toi *aussi* tu es capable de commencer quelque chose dans le monde, d'agir pour des raisons, de hiérarchiser tes préférences, de t'estimer les buts de ton action et, ce faisant, de t'estimer toi-même comme je m'estime moi-même."

[9] As Ricoeur says (1990, 223): "Dans la sympathie vraie, le soi, dont la puissance d'agir est au depart plus grande que celle de son autre, se retrouve affecté par tout ce que l'autre souffrant offer en retour. Car il procède de l'autre souffrant un donner qui n'est précisément plus puisé dans sa puissance d'agir et d'exister, mais dans sa faiblesse même."

# 3.

# *Democracy becomes care; Care becomes democracy*

Joan C. Tronto

In the "Summary of the Leading Issues" prepared for the seminar out of which this volume arises, two types of asymmetry are described: "the carereceiver's dependency o[n] caregivers," and "the lack of social esteem, self-esteem and payment of most caregivers." Further, since "care situations which exemplify inequalities, contrast with dominant values," the issue that was posed to the authors is this one: can *pitié*/compassion or *Anerkennung*/recognition help to provide a basis for counterbalancing such inequalities?

In order to answer this question, I would like to challenge some of the starting assumptions contained within this framing of the issues. I will argue that we need to be more specific about some realities of care before we can determine which philosophical conceptions might be useful to us. Not all care receivers are dependent, not all care providers are disregarded in society; the arrows of care dependence can point in both directions. While *pitié* and *Anerkennung* are helpful concepts to use in thinking about care, they are not, by themselves, sufficient to overcome the biases that create asymmetry in care. Furthermore, not all care is asymmetrical, and perhaps we make an error when we use asymmetrical care as our model. Indeed, we can make care considerably more equal if we change our starting assumptions about the nature of care. And I shall further argue that unless we place care into a *democratic*, *political* context, we cannot resolve these or other dilemmas about caring.

Asymmetry in care becomes a problem when we fail to see how profoundly care is reciprocal and therefore social. Every human is at once always a receiver of care, even as any of us are providers of care for others. This is so because every day, each person needs to meet both his or her basic physical needs and culturally constructed needs for decent lives. Because we live in a culture that begins from the self and its agency as the starting point for philosophical reflection, we are more likely to see the activities of care giving than care receiving as definitive. Many adults provide mostly self-care for themselves. But this is care, nonetheless. What happens when we begin to understand how thoroughly we are also care receivers, dependent upon the care given to us by ourselves and others? When we understand care in this way, the problem of care asymmetries looks different.

Humans are mortal; thus each human life is ultimately tragic. Our needs can never be completely met by ourselves or by others. And yet despite these ultimate limits, each of us cares for, and is cared for by, others. Often such care relations create imbalances which, again tragically, may not be brought back into balance within our lives. Relations of care are likely to be asymmetrical in several ways: sometimes the care-receiver is deeply dependent upon the care-giver; often, caregivers lack social esteem, self-esteem, and remuneration for their services.[1] How serious is this imbalance as a problem in social theory? If care is necessarily asymmetrical, what are the implications of this reality for the prospect of genuinely democratic societies? Further, since "care situations which exemplify inequalities, contrast with dominant values," the issue that is posed to us is this one: can compassion (*pitié*) or recognition (*Anerkennung*) help to provide a basis for counterbalancing such inequalities? In this essay, I shall disagree with some of the others in this volume and argue that neither compassion nor recognition is sufficiently relational to address the nature of care within the context of a democratic society. An alternative conception of care, one which draws upon attentiveness, responsibility, and responsiveness, better describes care. In so doing, I shall also argue that the proper context in which to think about care relationally must be as broad as our notion of society. In this way, the asymmetric problems of care can be best mitigated only politically, that is, in a society committed to democratic caring.

## 1. Defining care

Conventional accounts of care all begin from the perspective of the caregiver. As a result, all of these definitions miss something important about the nature of care, since care is always *also the activity of receiving care*. Indeed, the notion that reception can be active rather than passive already begins to undo our logics of action and passion; but it is important in solving the problem of asymmetric care to consider this point.

There is no consensus about the meaning of care. For some, care is always a dyad of care between one more powerful care-giver and a second weaker carereceiver (Noddings 1984). Scholars define care in a number of ways, but for most scholars, care is the "labor of love" in which private or intimate activity is performed in a particular emotional state. For example, Francesca Cancian follows the pioneering British sociologists, Janet Finch and Dulcie Groves, in offering this account:

> My working definition of care is: a combination of feelings of affection and responsibility, with actions that provide for an individual's personal needs or well-being in a face-to-face interaction. (Cancian 2000)

Such a definition has both strengths and weaknesses. Among its strengths are that it combines care as a disposition and an action. Nevertheless, there are also a number of problems with such a definition. It presumes that care is only the activity of individuals directed toward other individuals. Not only does this exclude care for the self, but it also excludes the possibility that institutions or groups of individuals can care, or that people can care from a distance. These possibilities are included in our everyday use of the language of care, and there are good reasons to include them.

Such a definition of care also excludes "bad care" from being care at all. Imagine a nursing home attendant who hates the patients and only performs her work in the most desultory fashion in order to avoid being fired and to collect her pay. Surely such a person is "caring," though not well. Thus building in affection and responsibility prejudge the quality of care.

The contrasting broad definition I shall use and defend was worked out by Berenice Fisher and me in 1990:

> a species activity that includes everything that we do to maintain, continue, and repair our 'world' so that we can live in it as well as possible. That world includes our bodies, our selves, and our environment, all of which we seek to interweave in a complex, life-sustaining web (Fisher and Tronto 1990).

And, when we are concerned with trying to discern how the care perspective might develop into a vision for political change, it probably makes sense that we begin with this broadest definition and work our way back to see whether it is incompatible with other accounts.

Fisher and I also described four phases of care; I later added moral dimensions to each of these phases: caring about, caring for, care giving, and care receiving. Caring about involves recognizing the need for care in the first place. It requires the special moral quality of attentiveness, of recognizing needs. Caring for involves assumption of responsibility for the caring work that needs to be done; its obvious moral corollary is responsibility. Care giving is the actual work of care. To it, I attach the *moral* quality of competence, which though often presumed to be a technical matter, is also well understood, I believe, as a moral category. Care receiving is the response of the thing cared for. It is not the sole duty of the cared-for, as for example in Nel Noddings' definition, but requires that all involved in the care process revisit the question of how well the care process has worked. Its moral quality is responsiveness. Fisher and I also noted that care can be provided in the household, in social institutions, and through market mechanisms.

This definition confounds many ways that social scientists divide their disciplines and perspectives; care for the self seems a psychological category, care for others a sociological category, care for the "world" economic and political categories. Further, this definition seems to combine normative standards ("as well as possible") with non-normative concerns, though it still allows us to adjudge some "caring" as bad care; it is not excluded by definition. This definition points to the advantages of a holistic over an analytical approach; for example, while "responsibility" is a part of the entire process of care, it is possible to imagine it absent from a particular care act (this nurse's aide only provides the medications because she was handed this cup of pills and told to dispense them). From this framework, then, care is not only something that we can measure by "the importance of what we care about..." nor is it reducible to an attitude of "thrownness," "altruism," alterity, compassion, recognition, etc. Care is about such attitudes, but it is also about taking responsibility, about doing well the work of care, and about responding to the needs for care that we have tried to meet. Care is also as much about receiving care as giving care, and the steps of attentiveness and responsiveness require that care be understood not only from the standpoint of the acting care-giver but from the acting care-receiver.

When we define care in this way, our world view changes. Suddenly, we do not only see the world as consisting of autonomous individuals pursuing rational ends and life projects, but we see the world as comprised of people enmeshed within networks of care and committed to meeting the caring needs around them. This is not to say that every activity in the world is care, but many activities are caring. And caring activities might turn out to be "nested" in the sense that they are pursued in order that they may contribute to achieving other ends. It is because we "nest" self-care so low in our daily pursuits that we forget to see it as care. This complex account of care is often simplified in order to make discussions of care simpler. But when we try to bracket this complexity, we often end up distorting the nature of care.

## 2. Problems with compassion and recognition

Both compassion and recognition are ultimately unable to help us to address the asymmetries of care because they start from the assumption of the agent/subject as a way to think about care. In the end, because they in part exempt the subject from the problem to be addressed, they are unable to create the complex interaction needed to resolve the problem of asymmetry.

Consider Housset's account of compassion (Housset 2003). Housset is trying to find a way to describe a pre-egoistic form of attachment to others. For Housset, compassion is not a voluntary act, nor the product of a decision. It is an encounter with the flesh of another person, something immediate and yet distant. The person who is compassionate is no longer a being with a conscience. The compassionate person is seeking to liberate him or herself from the abstraction of a closed world.[2] But such a form of compassion can only exist in a person who, has at least for the moment, surrendered the capacity for action and judgment. While in that moment, it is possible to escape from the sense of the deeply dependent one-cared-for as other, how can that form of compassion inform asymmetrical care once one comes back into the worlds of judgment and action? Housset's notion of compassion warns us against an overly instrumental account of others, and against objectifying others. But what stops us from engaging in such processes? Even if we are able to recapture the moment of compassion, how can it inform our actions?

Conceptions of recognition, on the other hand, are often highly rational. For Charles Taylor (1994), Axel Honneth (1996), and Nancy Fraser (1997; 2005), leading thinkers about the notion of recognition, the process of recognizing the other is an exercise of a kind of reason. For Taylor, recognition is the proper corrective to the misunderstandings of others that arise across cultural differences. Thus, he argues, "misrecognition shows not just a lack of due respect. It can inflict a grievous wound, saddling its victims with a crippling self-hatred. Due recognition is not just a courtesy we owe people. It is a vital human need." (Taylor 1994, 26) In introducing the language of "need," Taylor seems to be speaking about an approach compatible with an ethic of care. But the problem is that recognition is, for Taylor, a response to a previous injury, i.e., misrecognition. But there is nothing inherent in asymmetries of care to suggest that they require or signify misrecognition. As Kelly Oliver observes, in order for there to be recognition, there has had to be mis-recognition before it; in order to right an injustice, there is an assumption that injustice has already occurred (Oliver 2001, 48-49).[3] But, there is no "backstory" in Taylor, Honneth, or Fraser that explains how the misrecognition occurred in the first place. As Oliver points out, this failure to recognize the situatedness of the origin of the problem is already a serious problem in coming to any resolution of the problem. There is no dialectic in recognition; it is one-sided and, unlike Housset's notion of compassion, never requires the subject to leave her/his subjectivity aside. It does not require that the person who is "recognizing" sees him or herself reciprocally as requiring the recognition of the other.

There is a further danger here with theories of recognition as well; let me call it the "synecdoche" problem. It is that those who seek recognition because they have been misrecognized are often reduced, constantly, to the very difference that distinguishes them from those who misrecognize them. This problem is a familiar one within the discourses of identity politics; as the Afrian-American poet Pat Parker wrote to whites who would befriend her, "The first thing you do is to forget that i'm Black./ Second, you must never forget that i'm Black." (Parker 2000) Hence, gays are reduced to their sexuality, and, I shall argue later in this essay, "multicultural" people are increasingly reduced to their capacities as caregivers. Nancy Fraser herself identifies a version of this problem; she wants to avoid, she says, "reification" of the categories of identity (see Swanson 2005). But such reification is for Fraser an *intellectual* error, not a *relational* one. It is the fault of the *logic* (or the real world processes that Fraser sees resulting from such a logic) of requiring identity be recognized, not the fault of *the recognizer*. From the standpoint of a person whose need for care marks them as in an asymmetrical relationship of care, the solution of "recognition" simply reinscribes the perceived difference. While recognition is an attempt at an ethical solution, it is, in the end, unsatisfying.

Interestingly, then, Housset's conception of compassion is beneficial for solving this problem because of its immediacy; it works to eliminate judgment and thus to overcome asymmetry in that manner. The problem with the concept of recognition is that while it is a well-formed judgment, it is apt to distort the person's actual lived experience in the process of turning it into this judgment. Each could be a corrective for the other, except that they seem to pose the inadequacy of the other as a fundamental flaw. Neither alone nor together, then, do compassion and recognition solve the problem of asymmetrical relations of care.

If neither compassion nor recognition work as solutions to this problem, in what ways might we think that care can solve this problem? Indeed, if we accept the premise that we should care in ways that enhance democracy, then we notice instantly the problem that care creates for democracy: many care relationships are not relationships of equality. Humans are not equal in their capacities, especially if we include those who are too young, too infirm, too frail, within the society. Historically, democratic theorists and democratic practices solved this problem by excluding those who were "dependent" or not fully rational from being citizens. For the ancients, these exclusions extended to slaves and women. In the modern period, the struggles of democratic societies have been to expand those who are included as full citizens; property-less and working class men, and eventually women, were added to the franchise. But in a way, by leaving care behind the wall created through a rigid modern separation of public and private life, democratic societies continue to practice a kind of exclusion. Simply shutting the door on the modern, private, household, however, is no way to solve the problem of inequality. In this way, indeed, including care within the purview of the activities, concerns, and life of democratic citizens, really represents the next (perhaps last) frontier for democratic theory. Let us consider, then, some realities of care in contemporary democratic societies with an eye to addressing how a care perspective might aid in solving the problems asymmetrical care.

## 3. Some care realities

### *Necessary care and personal service: power and care relationships*

At the beginning, we should note that many care relations are asymmetrical, but not all of them are asymmetrical in the same direction.

Kari Waerness distinguishes among types of care; she includes these two: necessary care and personal service (Waerness 1990). Necessary care is care that one cannot provide for oneself, i.e., it requires the care of another. Personal service is care that one can provide for oneself, but chooses not to provide for oneself. The difference here is not about expertise, but about one's capacity to fulfill one's own needs. Thus, a brain surgeon provides necessary care, but a 12-year old neighbor who watches the baby for a few minutes does so as well (since the baby cannot watch itself). A launderer who is hired to clean one's clothes provides a personal service, but so too does a gourmet chef in a restaurant (since one can prepare one's own food, even if not so expertly). What is interesting to me about this difference, though, is to notice the different positions of power of the care givers and care receivers in the two situations. In the first, the care givers are more powerful because the care receivers are in need of their care—with many care givers, their care is vital for the life of the care receiver. In the second, though, the asymmetric arrow points the other way—and if the launderer fails to satisfy the demands of the care receivers for whatever they deem to be first rate service, she is likely to be fired. Because care work is often viewed as unskilled, its value is low and the service demanders are able to command their providers in highly asymmetric ways. (While I have somewhat stretched this distinction, and clearly there are exceptions, the point is that care and service may involve many of the same tasks: cleaning the body, the environment, repairing and sustaining damaged bodies and goods, but they are different in terms of the power dimensions of the relationships).

This distinction is important because it has several political implications. First, the boundary between necessary care and personal service will often be a *political* one. Consider the case of day care. If we think of the baby sitter as providing a *service* to the mother, then it is a service that is provided, and despite its necessity, the babysitter is not well compensated.[4] On the other hand, if we make a societal decision that day-care for young children is essential to fostering democratic values, then we might pay such teachers of children more than we currently do. Second, the phenomenon of "privileged irresponsibility," that some people can excuse themselves from care work because others will do it for them, fits nicely the logic of service. Third, if we confuse care and service we provide a way to separate democratic citizens from "needy" others in society. While all humans need care, if we think of care as service then we have a way to deny the centrality of care as a part of our human experience. We can then entertain the fantasy that we are not care-givers only because there are other more important things for "us" to do. We can entertain the fantasy, as able-bodied, rational, democratic citizens, that we do not receive care ourselves (even from ourselves). If we think of care as simply a convenience for others as it is for ourselves, then those who *really* need care must, by that need, disqualify themselves from citizenship and full participation in society. Thus, some democratic thinkers have argued that caring societies must only be sure about "protecting the vulnerable" (Goodin 1985). But this process sets up the "vulnerable" as different from, and incapable of, citizenship. And it allows society to treat care workers as expendable or low-skilled. Thus, care, though vital for our lives, becomes devalued in the economy and in the polity.

### *Of dyads and dualisms*

Nel Noddings famously described care as a dyad between care giver and care receiver, and for Noddings, no care existed unless the care receiver acknowledged the care received. The more I think about this question, not only is this model limited, it is completely wrong. There is no such thing as "Robinson Crusoe" care. We commit a grave ideological error if we use this metaphor to describe care.

Think of some cases of supposedly dyadic care: the doctor/patient relationship, the mother/child relationship, the teacher/student relationship. Doctors do not provide health care alone. They are increasingly involved in a complex set of social relationships of care. Families provide much of the health care that people receive. But other professionals, insurance companies, government agencies, hospital administrators, etc. etc. are also involved in care relations. To think of this as dyadic is obviously inaccurate. The same holds true with mother/child relationships. Although there is often a particularly strong bond between mothers and children, the ideological construction of this as the primary relationship of life is relatively new. In centuries past in western societies, children were sent to wet-nurses who might be some distance from their mother. The Doulia described by Eva Kittay is a helper who is present in the home early in the child's life. Nurse maids, fathers, siblings, grandparents, and other adults in the family are often significant influences in children's lives. The idea that only the mother cares for a child helps to create a misimpression about the nature of care. Similarly, while students learn from teachers, they do not only learn from teachers, nor do they mainly do so dyadically; little teaching is one-to-one.

Val Plumwood, in her important book on *Feminism and the Mastery of Nature*, (Plumwood 1993) warned us that when we create a dualism, often what we are trying to do is to cut off, dominate, cut out, the parts of the dominant reflected in the subordinate. In the "backgrounding," process, problematic qualities of the dominant which (even though they are present) are assigned to the subordinate. Hence, the dyad care-giver/care-receiver is not simply an analytical tool, it is also a way to avoid seeing that care givers too are also vulnerable, needy, incompetent. Many feminist scholars have written about the difficulties of "evidence blindness" (e.g. Hawkesworth 2006). Evidence blindness is another problem in asymmetrical care, in which the view of the care giver substitutes for the somewhat obvious evidence that the care receiver has a different perspective. Plumwood's notion of the backgrounding that results from dualism helps us to explain how this mechanism of "evidence blindness" functions. When a caregiving self cuts qualities out of the self and projects them on to the the care receiver, the resulting care is going to be distorted.

## 4. Some implications of these care realities

These care realities are deeply disturbing for any number of reasons, but let me highlight a few of them. First, the dyadic model of care serves to heighten our sense of "dis-ease" and discomfort about asymmetries of care. Within the framework of the dyad, the problems of asymmetries of necessary care are simply irresolvable. Even Noddings seems to notice this, stipulating that the care receiver must acknowledge the support, i.e., must be grateful. But the problem with this model is that it begins to import into the very nature of care its inequality. From the standpoint of democratic societies, such inequality can serve as a justification for continuing to exclude and not think about care receivers and their close care givers as full participating citizens.

Furthermore, the dyad keeps the focus always on the care-giver. We hardly ever think of ourselves as care-receivers. If "we" can be more compassionate, or exercise recognition, be better care-givers, then care will improve. But all of the focus is on the more powerful care-giver. Furthermore, the only possible agents for changing the situation are those who are already full participants. This is almost always a way in which those who are already more powerful are able to dismiss those they have made into "others."[5]

Thinking about such matters, I am lead to think of a care theorist's nightmare: that the distinction between care and service might become the distinction between "real care" and "commodity care." If care and service are close, then all care that is 'commodified' might come to be seen as service. This perception makes the care receiver more powerful. Starting from the premise of dyadic care, and if one is then concerned that there is an imbalance of power between care givers and care receivers, then this slide toward thinking of most care as service seems to a good step. It seems to suggest that there is a way to balance out the inequalities of care provision. It is a way to make care more "equal." (One version of this argument is to think of medical patients as "consumers.") Because it seems to solve one problem, it may be difficult to note that it creates many more problems.

The direction of the 'care drain' will make this transition from care to "commodity" easier. As care becomes more exclusively the work of "multiculturals", it will be easier to exclude them from citizenship. The public/private exclusion that has kept care out of private life might now become reinscribed as the care/service ground for exclusion. "Real care" will only be done by the unmarked, "original" people, while "service" will be marked by race, language, religion, migration status. Once this happens, it will be easy to return to a time before any assumptions about democratic equality prevailed. Susan Okin famously observed that political theory had always asked, "what are men like?" but "what are women *for*?" This question may switch its meaning, blunting feminist criticism, but making clear that what immigrants and people from other races and cultures are "for" is caring for "us."

Throughout the industrialized countries, for example, care workers are being imported, as care itself becomes a vital commodity (Parreñas 2001), yet at the same time, immigrants are vilified. In 2008 in Italy, days after he approved a "fast track" for immigrant home helps and carers, Welfare Minister Maurizio Sacconi stated that the Italian government is 'determined' to reduce the number of immigrants arriving in Italy (ANSA 2008; Corriere della Sera 2008). Immigrants are from this perspective seen not as people who have families, but people who can be exploited as workers. They are servants who enjoy what Parrenas has called "partial citizenship."

Can democracies survive if they transform some people into nothing but servants? Surely we can imagine such a social system; whether we can call it democratic is another issue.

## 5. Care and democracy

Perhaps we can stop this trend. To do so, we need to commit ourselves to make care a central value in democratic societies and to democratize care.

### *Care as a democratic value*

In order to make care a workable democratic value, we need to make certain our commitment to three sets of ideas.

1. *Care receivers all!* First, though some people are more vulnerable and dependent than others, we need to admit that we are all vulnerable.

Not only do I mean that each human began life as a helpless infant who needed the intensive care of many people, or that many of us will again become infirm or frail, but that each and every day we need care in order to sustain our lives. While many autonomous adults think that they care for themselves, in fact each of us is at the center of a complex web of relations of care. There is a continuum of how much care any one person needs, not a dichotomy between cared-for and care-giver.

This is not an easy idea for most people to endorse. It requires that we see ourselves as vulnerable. It requires that we surrender our senses of ourselves as entirely autonomous. And it requires that we stop thinking that "personal responsibility" is the solution to all problems of society. Indeed, a genuine recognition of our large and interrelated vulnerability may well change the way that we think about social responsibilities.

2. *Care about equality and equality of care.* Democratic societies will not succeed in remaining democratic for long if the imbalances of wealth and income persist. This is not only because there is a danger of becoming "dependent" upon those who are wealthy, or because (as social psychologists and political theorists correctly argue) we identify with the wealthy and are willing to accept their interests as ours. It is also because if resources for care are unequal, we will never be able to achieve the democratic goal of equal opportunity or what theorists of justice describe as open and fair competition for posts in society. Equal access to care well is as necessary as making certain that people have opportunities. Jody Heymann, an epidemiologist at Harvard University, argued that one of the qualities of being poor or working-class is that one has many fewer resources for caring well for one's children (Heymann 2000). As a result, the levels of inequality of care turn into inequalities of access to education, good jobs, and hence, to further economic equality. Poor parents have lives that do not permit them to care as well for their children as wealthy parents. If we do not notice this imbalance, then inequality will continue to grow.

3. *Care about plurality, otherness*. Care is universal, but how needs are shaped and met admit of great cultural variation. Democratic societies have an obligation to allow, protect, and indeed, to cherish, such variation. This does not mean that all cultural practices are permitted if they are called "caring," but it does provide the substantive focus around which such disputes might be shaped. Questions of equality are foremost for caring about democracy; so too must the treatment of cultural differences reflect a commitment to caring well in democratic ways.

### *Democratic care is best*

Finally (and here I provide my most direct response to the questions of how to solve the problems of asymmetries of care), care is better when done democratically. "Two heads are better than one," goes the saying in English. "Triangulation" is a more effective form of navigation and of research. The dyadic model of care is not only inaccurate, it is also normatively not a good model of care. Care, like other aspects of human life, benefits from being done by more people. While there is a limit to how large any given circle of care might expand, there are ways to try to insure that the circles of care are wide enough to guarantee that the quality of care will be well provided. Robert Helmreich and his team of researchers, for example, compared pilots and their training with doctors and their training (Sexton et al. 2000). They discovered that doctors are still trained more hierarchically and are more likely to think of errors as a personal responsibility. On the other hand, after carefully studying plane crashes, the trainers of pilots realized that if members of a crew deferred to the pilot's understanding of the situation, they were often unable to correct a mistake. Once pilots were trained to recognize that crews make mistakes, that mistakes are not a sign of weakness but are natural, they were able to work within a more flattened hierarchy to resolve problems more effectively. Flattening out hierarchies provided better opportunities to prevent serious errors. (Indeed, many utopian theories do not permit children to be raised by families.)

### *Starting from the needs of care receivers, thinking of rights and needs*

Care receivers have needs. They also have rights. It is important to think about both the needs of care receivers and their rights. The danger is that democratizing care may lead to a competition among needs, rather than a commitment on the part of society to address all of the needs that are urgent. In the USA and in other countries, governments sometimes create "block grants" to meet the needs of citizens, allowing states or localities to decide for themselves how to distribute inadequate resources. Advocates for care cannot allow such pitting of care needs against one another; this is the point at which a discourse of rights becomes vital.

### *The global scope of care provision and care crises.*

"Globalization" needs also to be understood from a care perspective. Care relations and responsibilities reach far beyond the family, town, and nation-state. Concrete anchors, such as human rights, can help guide us. But we have to be willing to care, support care, and receive care in turn.

If this sounds an echo, let it be Aristotle: a citizen is one who rules and is ruled in turn. So too citizens and global citizens need care and can care effectively for others in different degrees. While Aristotle thought it proper to exclude some in order to make this kind of reciprocity work, our greater powers to distribute resources, to care for people and the environment, create for us greater responsibilities. We have to accept these new responsibilities as the challenge that faces us. That is the promise of democratic care, and it is the only solution to our concerns about asymmetrical care.

## Notes

[1] See the introduction of this volume.

[2] My discussion of Housset owes a great deal to the explication of his ideas by Frans Vosman at the conference, and I am grateful for these discussions. See Housset in this volume.

[3] A similar point is made very well by Willett (2001).

[4] Some years ago, the *New York Times* ran an article in their consumer pages about hiring a nanny. "You want someone who puts the children before herself," said Judy Meyers, 37, a mother of two in Briarcliff Manor, N.Y., who works for a health insurance company. "But to find someone for the right amount of money is not so easy." (Rubenstein 1993)

[5] "Within the conjunction of disability as personal tragedy and bioethics as medical ethics, the presence of disability presents them as an anathema to the good…..These implicit and unquestioned understandings result in a relationship between bioethics and disability which is more likely to be focused upon the ethical practices of carers, practitioners, clinicians, technicians, and ethicists. It is their works which are assessed in light of assumed goodness, that is, for their capacity to normatively respond to the presumed themes of imbued unhappiness, suffering, burden, dependence, incompetence, undesirability, irrelevance and the need to control Dependent Others." (Clapton 2003, 542).

# 4.

# *Things to do with stories*

Hilde Lindemann

The picture of morality emerging from the grand moral theories developed by the philosophers of the Enlightenment—social contract theory, utilitarianism, and Kantian ethics—has been under siege for some time now. A number of moral theorists have rejected the idea that morality consists of a solitary judge applying law-like principles logically deduced from a comprehensive, impartialist, universalist moral theory to the specifics of an instant case. Bernard Williams (1981), for example, famously observed that the theoretically unlimited demands of impartialist systems of morality elbow out much that gives meaning to life, including anything that could inspire us to take any moral goal seriously. Michael Stocker (1987) criticized such systems on the grounds that their impersonal stance prevents them from capturing what is morally significant about such interpersonal relationships as friendship, love, or community. Feminist ethicists argued that the model's transcendental "view from nowhere" is actually a view from male privilege that fails to take women's interests and experiences seriously. Postmodernists challenged the model's representation of the moral subject as a unified self with a private, disembodied consciousness.

Two of the more interesting challenges to the Enlightenment model are moral particularism and the recent narrative turn in ethics. Moral particularism denies that any theory can generate code-like rules for assigning the correct moral valuation to natural properties, arguing that making moral judgments is more like getting a joke than like applying principles—every natural situation has its own particular properties and these come together in a kind of gestalt that lets you judge the situation as "cruel" or "murder," or "courageous." By the narrative turn in ethics I mean the variety of recent approaches that accord a central role to stories, not merely employing them to illustrate moral concepts such as justice or neighborly love, or to test our moral intuitions, but regarding them as necessary means to some moral end. In this chapter, I want to examine a number of claims that have been made in the last twenty years or so concerning the moral work that narratives are capable of—in particular, those that propose to unseat the Enlightenment model in favor of a unique narrative ethics. To organize the claims under examination, I'm going to take up, in turn, each of seven sorts of things that can be done with stories. The first thing we can do with stories is read them. Second, we can invoke them. Third, we can compare them. Fourth, we can construct them. Fifth, we can counter them. Sixth, we can analyze them. And seventh, we can parody them. After I've discussed the moral purposes to which each of these narrative acts can be put, I'll offer my own account of the differences between Enlightenment and narrative approaches to ethics.

## 1. The stories we read

The first thing we can do with stories is *read* them (or listen to them, or view them). Here the moral purpose is to attend carefully to the nuances and complexities of great literature, films, or plays as a means of broadening one's morally formative experiences and so sharpening one's moral sensibilities. Martha Nussbaum (1990) is perhaps best known for her exploration of the role of artistic literature in developing the moral emotions. By reading serious fiction, she argues, one can make of oneself a person "on whom nothing is lost." One does this by allowing the author of the work to direct one's attention to the rich and subtle particulars of the narrative—the moral, intellectual, emotional, and social nuances. When the author has set these out with skill and imagination, overlooking no meaningful detail, the educated reader can see what is morally at issue in the narrative: she becomes, in the words Nussbaum borrows from Henry James, "finely aware and richly responsible." "Moral knowledge," Nussbaum writes, "is not simply intellectual grasp of propositions; it is not even simply intellectual grasp of particular facts; it is perception. It is seeing a complex, concrete reality in a highly lucid and richly responsive way; it is taking in what is there, with imagination and feeling" (Nussbaum 1990, 152). Having broadened her field of vision and refined her moral perception, Nussbaum argues, the reader is in a better position to respond excellently to actual people in the world.

Any approach to ethics that centers on the stories we read, though, raises the question of *what* to read. In his book *Balance and Refinement* (1993), Michael DePaul tells a story that illustrates this problem nicely. He imagines a naïve young man named Billy who, realizing that he is sexually inexperienced, decides to read novels for the purpose of cultivating a fine-grained moral response to some future soul mate. But he makes a serious blunder. He picks up a bodice-ripper on the way out of the supermarket, really likes it, and starts to form the impression that women like to be swept off their feet by manly men and enjoy being overpowered even to the point of rape. Billy knows he can't overcome his naiveté by reading only one novel, so he continues to broaden his experience with more literature of the same kind. But because he has so little experience of real women, the only fiction that rings true to him is the kind that endorses the "treat 'em rough" school of thought he first encountered at the supermarket. And then we can imagine that the same holds for his personal life: the relationships with women that he finds the most satisfying are the ones that conform to his favorite depictions of sweet savage love. "The end result of the whole affair," DePaul remarks sadly, "is that Billy's moral judgments regarding appropriate relations between men and women are thoroughly fouled up."

The trouble with Billy isn't just that he's sexually incompetent. He's *narratively* incompetent, and that might be what's gotten him into his present predicament. Narrative competence may be defined, first, as the ability to *choose* good literature, and second, as the ability to *read* good literature with care, skill, and critical judgment. It's the capacity for selecting works of fiction that are worth one's time and attention, and then reading these works shrewdly, with an awareness of the literary techniques the author employs and a sense of how the text relates to other literary texts. It involves knowing the standards for what makes a work of literary art good or great and either using those standards to evaluate what one reads or calling them into question.

But is it the lack of this sort of knowledge that has fouled up Billy's relations with the opposite sex? Note that the relevant standards are primarily *aesthetic* ones—the ones we use for judging literature as a work of art. If I am trying to refine my *moral* perception, though, why should those be the right standards? Mightn't it be more important for me to learn how to choose books—even books of poor literary quality—that can improve my moral position, and then learn how to read these books in ways that make me a morally better person? If choosing and reading books for these purposes involve standards other than aesthetic ones, then attaining *narrative* competence won't help me become "richly responsible."

Suppose that before Billy's fateful day at the supermarket he had gone to Nussbaum to ask her what he should read, and she advised him to pick a novel that people with highly developed levels of narrative competence have found worthy. Odd advice, he might think to himself. He might well wonder what narratively competent people know about love that he doesn't. He's probably met literary scholars who are just as naive about relationships with women as he is—and if he hasn't, I have. The English professor who is a renowned Shakespeare scholar but an inept human being doesn't read great authors with a view to her own moral improvement. She doesn't approach the texts in the right spirit, or use them for the purpose of cultivating her moral perception. Why, then, should her standards for good literature guide the naif's choice of what to read? Nussbaum clearly appreciates the importance of reading great literature in the proper frame of mind if one is to improve one's moral position. But the proper frame of mind has less to do with one's *narrative* competence than with one's *moral* competence, and about this the literary scholar, *qua* literary scholar, has no special expertise. If I'm right about the difference between the ability to read good literature and the ability to read literature in a way that makes you good, it turns out that narrative competence required for this approach is at best insufficient to the task of improving one's moral perception.

Proponents of the literary narrative approach are typically not so much interested in overthrowing the Enlightenment model as in refining the sensibilities of the inquirer who uses it. Nussbaum insists that "perceptions 'perch on the heads' of the standing terms; they do not displace them" (Nussbaum 1990, 155). There would be no conceptual incoherence in embracing the literary narrative approach while at the same time repudiating the Enlightenment model, but I'm not aware of any attempt to work out this position.

## 2. The stories we invoke

The second of the narrative approaches to ethics works with stories by *invoking* them. In a flat-out rejection of the Enlightenment model, Alasdair MacIntyre (1984) claims that reason and rationality are always characteristic of a specific historical tradition. It is the story of one's community—whether it be ancient Greece, medieval Paris, or eighteenth-century Edinburgh—that develops one's capacity to see things as reasonable, appropriate, valuable, and so on. Because the narrative tradition of the community subtly shapes all its members' knowing and valuing, there is no one model of moral reasoning that can be used as a vantage point from which to pass judgment on all the many cultures within which human beings live.

The Enlightenment model, taking itself to be precisely such a vantage point, is thus dismissed by the proponents of historical narrative as a philosophical cul-de-sac, a dead hope. In its place they call for an ethics based on what might be called the "just-so" stories of a culture: like Rudyard Kipling's stories of how the elephant got his trunk or the camel his hump, the high mythical and historical narratives of our communities explain who we are as a people and how we came to be this particular "we." These foundational narratives serve as the community's source of moral normativity, and we invoke them as a means of ethical justification. When we have run out of reasons for acting as we do, we appeal to the norms that are internal to the social practices of the community—norms which are in turn justified by the community's "just-so" stories. So, to take an obvious example, physicians might look to the history of medicine and the physician's traditional role in society as justification for refusing to participate in physician-assisted suicide: the norms internal to the practice of medicine forbid physicians to kill their patients, and the rightness of these norms is explained by invoking the foundational story of the Hippocratic tradition.

The advantages of invoking a culture's stories are evident: it generates an ethics that is much more useful for guiding action than are the transcendental principles of the Enlightenment model. A complaint commonly lodged against Kantian ethics, for example, is that any maxim to be universalized in accordance with the Categorical Imperative must be couched at such a high level of abstraction that it can't tell us what we ought to do in a given set of circumstances, but only (sometimes) what we mustn't do (Nussbaum 1992). The corresponding complaint against utilitarian ethics is that its prescriptions, when they aren't platitudes, are often counterintuitive or hopelessly vague. They depend heavily on uncertain predictions and interpersonal comparisons of utility that are difficult to make (Williams 1981). On the historical approach, by contrast, one need merely invoke one's story to find the rationale for one's action.

However, the drawbacks to the approach are perhaps as obvious as its merits. For one thing, in many communities, including the United States and Canada, the "just-so" stories forcibly include and oppress certain people at the same time as they exclude and silence certain others. "Our" culture's traditions aren't apt to yield a picture of the good life that could ever be adopted by those who find themselves on the margins of the culture, or those who are subordinated within the culture. This use of narrative unjustly excludes certain people from the community altogether, while at the same time it problematically includes certain other people by characterizing their lives within the community as unsuccessful or fit only for others' purposes. And what of people within the culture whose positions are liminal? What, for example, of the Capulet in love with the Montague, the person of mixed race, the transgendered person? How are *they* to understand themselves with respect to the community's traditions?

If the historical narrative approach is fraught with problems of inclusion and exclusion *within* a community's traditions, it is also at a disadvantage when it comes to reconciling the traditions *between* communities. As John Arras has pointed out, "foundational stories not only tell us who we are; they also tell us who we are not" (Arras 1997, 75). As a community, we define ourselves against other communities, positioning ourselves as not-Protestant if we are Catholic, not-Palestinian if we are Israeli. Often, these "not" relationships involve the domination of the one over the other, and usually this Other figures in the community's foundation myths as an objectified element rather than a subject community with myths of its own. So, as Arras points out,

> for contemporary Palestinians the relevant story is the history of their oppression at the hands of the Jewish state; conversely, for contemporary Israelis the relevant foundational story is the history of Palestinian aggression and terrorism. The subjects of these historical narratives are thus locked in a perpetual struggle, not only over land, but also over the meaning of their common history (75).

When cultures clash and traditions are at odds, the exhortation to invoke one's own tradition offers no political or moral relief. If the impasse is to be resolved peacefully, each side will likely have to make an effort to hear and understand the other's story. Often, such efforts fail or never get off the ground, but supposing the parties did somehow manage to hear one another, it's possible that they might come to question their own stories as a result, and then they would need some standard for judging which story is better—or indeed, whether either story is morally adequate. Invoking their own tradition to settle the dispute won't help, for that is to use as a yardstick the very thing that one is trying to measure.

MacIntyre (1988) refuses to give up on narrative in his attempt to solve the problem of competing stories. He claims that some new stories do a better job than the old ones of solving the problems that prompted people to call the old stories into question in the first place. When members of a narrative tradition come to see the tradition as ultimately unable to resolve its problems, the tradition experiences an "epistemological crisis" (361) for which its resources are no longer adequate. At that point, says MacIntyre, the members may look to outside traditions to show them not only a new set of social roles and new narratives to justify them, but also a way out of the crisis. MacIntyre insists that the adoption of new stories constitutes epistemological and moral progress. The new story is *better* than the old at solving the problems set for it—"better" according to the evaluative standards inherent in the old narrative tradition—so we haven't settled for a mere succession of one story after another. In this way, he claims, the historical narrative approach to ethics can remain critical without ultimately abandoning narrative for transcendental principles.

MacIntyre's solution may well be the right one, especially when one considers that the evaluative standards inherent in any tradition are often at odds with one another, such that a new story can appeal to norms that were present but not taken seriously enough in the old ways of understanding the tradition. The sticking-point, however, is MacIntyre's failure to recognize that disenfranchised or subordinated members of the community were in epistemological crisis *all along*. They can't rely on the modes of thought and evaluation made available by the tradition, because they are either alienated from those modes or connected to them in morally troublesome ways. This is not to say that they can't at all draw on the resources implicit in the standing narratives. But it does mean that they have to approach those narratives with suspicion and distrust, and that they must continually challenge their authority. Once it's acknowledged that the normativity of the "just-so" stories must be called into question by some of the community's members all of the time, and by all of the community's members in times of crisis, we have a more complicated picture than the one MacIntyre offers us of how stories perform the work of moral justification.

The method of invoking stories, then, is a repudiation of the Enlightenment model of morality. That model offers us a picture of morality that is atemporal and transcendental, and it's precisely these features of the model that MacIntyre rejects. The invocation of the historical narratives of one's culture to explain what we do and who we are presupposes a historically particular and culturally specific moral epistemology—the antithesis of the Enlightenment's insistence on one rationality that is everywhere and at all times the same.

### 3. The stories we compare

The third approach is to *compare* a story that is morally puzzling to a paradigm story or stories whose moral meaning is clear. The paradigm story, according to proponents of casuistry, displays summaries of shared moral understandings that are already embedded in our actual practices, and these summaries serve as action-guiding principles. Thus, when we come across a new case that leaves us uncertain how to proceed, we can look to the paradigm case for guidance.

The principles displayed by the paradigm case are always subject to revision in light of new cases. This is so not only because casuistical principles are derived from practice (they emerge from the 'bottom up' rather than being applied from the 'top down,' as on the Enlightenment model), but because discerning just which particulars of a story are morally relevant is a messy and uncertain business, and may require a number of passes before we get it right. As subsequent cases reveal new implications of principles embedded in the paradigm case, our view of the paradigm case may shift, causing us to modify our understanding of the original principles or perhaps even to replace them with new principles altogether. As Arras puts it, "Casuistical analysis might be summarized as a form of reasoning by means of examples that always point beyond themselves. Both the examples and the principles derived from them are always subject to reinterpretation and gradual modification in light of subsequent examples" (Arras 1991, 35-36).

One of the advantages of the casuistical approach to ethics is that our society is familiar with this form of reasoning: it's how judges, lawyers, and juries in the U.S. and other English-speaking countries build the body of common law. A second advantage is that the stories we compare, like the stories we invoke, are much better at telling the inquirer just exactly what she ought to do than is the Enlightenment model. But whereas the stories we invoke are a community's morally problematic "just-so" stories, casuistry makes use of more local and more easily revisable stories that needn't exclude or subordinate anybody.

Still, the method has its disadvantages. For one thing, some of its proponents claim that the work of comparing cases for moral guidance requires no theoretical apparatus, which seems to be a claim that the stories speak for themselves. They don't, of course. If Thomas Kuhn and other philosophers are right to argue that all perception is theory-laden, then so is the perception of events and circumstances that constitute a case. The particulars that are selected out of the manifold of experience for inclusion in the case are chosen according to some theory about their relevance to the story. Moreover, the instant case is compared to the paradigm case on the basis of some theory about the relationship between the two. This means that theoretical disagreements can arise not only about what facts are morally salient in the instant case, but also about whether an analogy actually exists between an instant case and any particular paradigm case.

But notice that the kind of theory needed here isn't necessarily what the Enlightenment philosophers meant by 'theory.' There, the theory is comprehensive, and meant to yield lawlike principles for guiding action or assessing situations. Here, the theory is local and restricted in scope, with much more modest ambitions. Comparing stories as a method of moral deliberation can therefore be seen as a way of parting company with the Enlightenment model of morality.

## 4. The stories we construct

The fourth approach is to *construct* stories—stories of personal identity. Marya Schechtman has usefully distinguished between two senses of identity. The first has to do with the question of whether a person at one point in time is still the same as the person at an earlier point in time. Call this the reidentification question. The second has to do with how the person sees herself and who other people understand her to be. In this sense of personal identity, the question isn't "Am I still the same person?" but "Who am I?" Call this the characterization question (Schechtman 1996).

I have argued elsewhere (Nelson 2001) that personal identities in the sense of the characterization question are narratively constituted. They consist of tissues of stories and fragments of stories, generated from both first- and third-person perspectives, that cluster around what we take to be our own or others' most important acts, experiences, characteristics, roles, relationships, and commitments. In short, they are narrative understandings formed out of the interaction between one's self-concept and others' sense of who one is. And because stories depict time passing, the narratives that constitute identities can reflect the respects in which we change, as well as how we remain the same.

Many of the narrative understandings forming a part of a personal identity draw on stock plots and character types that are familiar to us all. At some point in your life, perhaps, you might have understood your relationship with a lover by configuring it according to the stock boy-meets-girl script that structures everything from "Cinderella" to *Chicken Run*; the story then becomes a piece of your identity-constituting autobiography. A friend betrays you and you identify him in biblical terms: he is a Judas. A white police officer sees a black teenager driving his mother's BMW and pigeonholes him as a drug dealer or a car thief, drawing on the representations of African American youths that saturate the media. Socially shared narratives like these contribute to the identities of groups as well as individuals, and members of the group draw a part of their identity from how the group identity is narratively constructed.

Other parts of the narrative tissue that constitute a personal identity consist of the localized, particular stories that pick an individual out as distinct from others in the groups to which she belongs: these are the stories that distinguish, say, your grandmother from the other members of her family, or from the class of grandmothers in general. They are the stories of your grandmother's arrival in this country from Germany after the First World War, of the vacations you spent with her when you were young, of the yearly excursions when she would take you out into the woods to show you where the earliest spring flowers grew, and of how consistently and hilariously she used to mangle the English language.

Personal identities function as counters in our social transactions, in that they convey understandings of what those who bear them are expected to do. If an answer to Who are you? is "the bartender," for example, I expect you to know how to mix a Manhattan; if the answer is "Arthur Frank," I don't. Moreover, identities also stand surrogate for how those who bear them may be treated. If you're my three-year-old son, I can remind you to use the toilet, but if you're my boss, I'd better not. Personal identities make intelligible to us, then, not only how other people are supposed to act, but how *we* are supposed to act with respect to them.

From a first-person perspective, personal identities function in much the same way. I treat myself with contempt or respect depending on who I think I am, and out of that narratively constructed sense of myself I also establish certain expectations for how I ought to behave in the future. But the fit between my identity and my agency goes in both directions: if it's true that I act out of the tissue of stories that constitute my sense of who I am, it's just as true that I express who I am by how I act. In fact, my actions are important criteria for assessing the accuracy of my self-conception. If, for instance, I see myself as a good driver but I've received four traffic citations in the last six months, others have reason to doubt, in this respect, at any rate, that my identity-constituting stories are credible ones.

As the good driver example reveals, personal identities may be sites of contestation. This is particularly true for members of minority groups who have been persistently misidentified by those in the dominant culture. So, for example, the black teenager driving his mother's BMW doesn't at all view himself the way the racist white cop does.

In his case, the difference of opinion over who he is can, although perhaps with difficulty, be resolved, as soon as his mom comes down to the station house to set the officer straight. In other cases, recognition of a self-understanding may be impossible to come by, because the person lacks the social standing that permits her own story about who she is to be taken up by others.

The stories we construct allow us to represent people in their particularity rather than in the generalities required by the Enlightenment model. For that reason, although it's not incompatible with it, I'm inclined to set story construction outside the theoretical-juridical moral framework.

## 5. The stories we counter

Sometimes we find that we need to convince others that we are responsible, morally upright, trustworthy people. One way of doing this is to *counter* the story of who they take us to be. This use of stories has close affinities with story construction, because it's the stories we construct to form our self-conception that we act out of when we need to persuade others to change their minds about who we are. To show you what I mean, let me recount a story Gareth Williams tells about one woman's interaction with the British National Health Service. According to Williams, the Thatcher administration, whose reigning tactic was to blame the poor for their poverty and the ill for their illness, invoked the Calvinistic "just-so" stories of Protestantism in support of the view that health is a matter of right conduct, while illness is a sign of sinfulness and a warning to amend one's ways. Mrs. Fields, an impoverished sixty-two-year-old widow with acute rheumatoid arthritis, purposefully repudiated this characterization. Keenly aware of the stories by which the government constructed the identities of people like her, she developed a counterstory whose aim was to shift how the representatives of the National Health Service viewed her. She acted out, for the district nurse, her own sense of who she was, deliberately and conscientiously remaining physically independent, staying out of debt, and keeping her house clean. She proudly told Williams,

> The other week, the district nurse came running in saying, "Do you mind if I use your toilet?" Now the first thought in my mind was, "She's a nurse, they're particular, she wouldn't ask to go to my toilet if I was dirty." You know, you think you've achieved something. I know it may sound simple to you, but it's not. That was something important. She can't think I'm careless, and she's not frightened of touching anything in the house.

The stories we enact to counter the stories that have stereotyped us in morally degrading ways can have their own drawbacks, however. Mrs. Fields's story of independence, cleanliness, and financial responsibility allowed her to resist being seen as just another drain on the National Health. But she only constituted her *own* identity with this counterstory. Because her enactment left untouched the Calvinistic and Thatcherite narratives that the government used to constitute the identity of the other chronically ill people in her socioeconomic class, the counterstory identified Mrs. Fields as an *exception*. So while it allowed the district nurse to see her as a competent moral agent, it did nothing to reidentify the others who share her plight. A better story would have been one that repudiated Mrs. Thatcher's story altogether, as that might have repaired the damage done to the entire class of people who were too poor to pay for their own health care.

Mrs. Fields's story boomerangs back on the other members of her group, but that's only one way in which self-defining counterstories can misfire. Hostage stories are another: think of the counterstory circulating in the African American community that urges black men to take pride in their race by identifying themselves as manly, heterosexual men. In the words of gangsta-rapper Ice Cube, "true niggers ain't gay." This story counters racist oppression, all right, but it takes gays and lesbians hostage as it does so. The "we are who I am" story also misfires, because it overgeneralizes from a specific case. Here an example would be Betty Friedan's *The Feminine Mystique*, which takes the plight of bored suburban housewives as representative of the oppression of all women. When Friedan urges middle-class women to "hire a cleaning lady" and go out and get a career, it's clear that for her, cleaning women don't qualify as part of the "we" who need liberation. And finally, there's the bathwater story, which dislodges not only the oppressive identity it sets out to resist, but also other fundamental, shared understandings. I'm thinking in this connection of the counterstories that some disability rights activists construct to counter the stories that identify them almost solely in terms of their disability. One such counterstory represents disability as simply one more form of human variation, like eye color. But if, say, spina bifida were simply a neutral human variation, then it wouldn't make sense to expend significant social resources on surgical and other therapies to correct it, and there wouldn't be any reason for women to take folic acid during pregnancy to prevent the condition, unless they happened to prefer intact neural tubes for their children. Bathwater stories throw out too much—important moral responsibilities go down the drain right along with the narratives that need to be discarded.

Enacting a counterstory might be seen as compatible with the Enlightenment model of morality, because what the story counters is a social injustice which it would be wrong to inflict on anybody, anywhere. But the concept of justice needn't be thought of as a law-like principle wielded by a solitary judge, even in cases where we want to say that its scope is universal. We can conceive of justice instead as a flexible concept that takes on slightly different meanings in different contexts—here, as a way of marking something that is morally relevant to our understanding of the relationship between Mrs. Field and the National Health system. For that reason, I'd argue that an approach to ethics employing the stories we enact need not presuppose an Enlightenment view of morality.

### 6. The stories we analyze

A sixth approach to ethics is that of *literary analysis*. One of the more significant developments in literary criticism is the subfield of narratology, which developed as a reaction to structuralist linguistics. Structuralism offered formal, scientific accounts of the grammar and deep structure of language, based on differences in sound production that could be marked, mapped, and classified. Entertaining the possibility that narratives too might have a grammar and deep structure, Vladimir Porpp, Tzvetan Todorov, Claude Lévi-Strauss, Roland Barthes, and others applied structuralist methodology to folktales, films, and other narrative forms. But in the 1960s Jacques Derrida and others challenged the French structuralists' "lab coat" approach to literature, arguing that a purely formal system of linguistic differences can refer to nothing outside itself and so is incapable of anchoring meaning—and in particular, *moral* meaning. The earlier work of Mikhail M. Bakhtin now helped linguistic structuralism refocus on narrative's social dynamics: Bakhtin and Fredric Jameson, among others, offered powerful demonstrations of how the analysis of form could be used to critique social ideologies. This social critique now dominates narratology.

Literary theorists using the resources of narratology have analyzed stories from the perspectives of Marxism, feminism, and critical race theory to critique abusive group relations as they appear in literature, but they have also approached various social practices and other artifacts as if they were literary texts, analyzing them with the help of techniques of literary criticism. So, for example, Anne Hunsaker Hawkins has used James Joyce's concept of the "epiphany"—a sudden revelation of profound meaning—to describe an element in the way physicians perceive and resolve ethical issues.

While narratologists and proponents of ethical criticism are surely "doing ethics" as they "do stories," they are typically bringing moral resources to bear on narrative rather than the other way around. For that reason, the method requires a great deal of training and the cultivation of a number of scholarly skills. It's not a method for just anyone to use. In fact, if you aren't a trained literary scholar, don't try this one at home.

Using the tools of literary criticism to offer a moral analysis not only of a story but also of social practices *as* stories can certainly be done by drawing on the resources of the Enlightenment model of morality, but, as with those who enact counterstories, it needn't be. It all depends on what view the critic takes of moral theory.

## 7. The stories we parody

A final thing we can do with stories for moral purposes is to *parody* them. Here, for example, I am thinking of the culturally dominant stories we use to construct gender in our society. Stories such as "Snow White" teach little girls that they will find fulfillment in serving men, while teenage girls learn from any number of movies, commercials, and rock videos how to assume the persona of the sex goddess whose business it is to make men happy. In the mean time, adolescent boys learn from the narratives in video games that women exist to serve men sexually and can be blown away at will.

In *Gender Trouble*, Judith Butler points to the practices of drag, cross-dressing, and butch/femme stylizing for their ability to parody these depictions. Drag subverts the fiction of the womanly woman and the manly man, and it does it by exaggerating the dominant stories. Drag often involves cross-dressing, but not always. Greta Garbo, observes Parker Tyler,

> 'got in drag' whenever she took some heavy glamour part, whenever she melted in or out of a man's arms, whenever she simply let that heavenly-flexed neck . . . bear the weight of her thrown-back head. . . . How resplendent seems the art of acting! It is all *impersonation*, whether the sex underneath is true or not (Butler 1990, 128).

By the same token, Dolly Parton has made a lifelong career out of performing drag, while the famous cover photo for *Vanity Fair* in which a scantily clad Cindy Crawford gives K. D. Lang a shave features everybody in drag, though only Lang is cross-dressed. And the film *The Adventures of Priscilla, Queen of the Desert* parodies all sorts of dominant stories about sex, heterosexuality, and gender, as Terence Stamp imposes on his own performance of masculinity the role of a postsurgical male-to-female transsexual who performs as a gay drag queen and who, not as a gay man but as a woman, takes a male lover. Here the opportunities for parody are amazingly rich, as a man plays the role of a woman who used to be a man, playing the role of a man playing a woman. Parody can be put to a number of purposes, many of them nonmoral. But if Butler is right about drag, this kind of parody does the moral work of resisting oppressive stereotypes.

While parodies do perform a kind of *reductio ad absurdum* on stories that are less than socially desirable, they are not capable of showing us which stories fall under that category. They don't, in other words, show us what *ought* to be parodied. Nor do they provide us with the resources for constructing better stories. They show us what to avoid, but not where we ought to go instead.

As for their relationship to the Enlightenment model of morality, this could be perfectly straightforward, in that the model could easily be used to guide the choice of the story to be targeted. There are, for example, plenty of resources on the Enlightenment model to explain what's wrong with the depictions of women as men's sexual servants. On the other hand, the model could *itself* be the target. We can imagine parodies that mock the inadequacies of the Kantian or utilitarian way of thinking about morality—parodies that are employed by those who repudiate that model. As with the two previous methods, whether this one works with or against the Enlightenment model depends on what view the parodist takes of moral theory.

## 8. The moral work that stories do

Any judgment as to whether stories can do the various kinds of moral work that are claimed for them depends on what, precisely, one takes morality to be. The Enlightenment model represents morality as a codifiable set of moral formulas, typically conceptualized as rules or principles at a high level of generality, which any agent can apply to a situation to guide action or assess wrongdoing. On this model the (solitary) moral philosopher's task is to construct, test, and refine covering laws that exhibit moral knowledge. The task of moral justification is carried out by the covering principles or procedures that make up the moral theory.

On the Enlightenment model a story might instantiate a principle, but it's the principle, not the story, that justifies action. Stories could serve other purposes, though. For one thing, even the most ardent proponents of utilitarianism or social contract theory will acknowledge that most people learn most of what they know about morality from stories of one sort or another, beginning with nursery tales told to children just learning to talk. For another, on the Enlightenment model, stories might also serve as heuristic devices for the abstractly impaired—the people who lack the talent to grasp, or to learn how to use, the propositions that are the proper medium for moral reasoning.

Some of us who have lost faith in the Enlightenment model of morality, however, favor what Margaret Urban Walker has dubbed an expressive-collaborative view of morality. On this model, morality is something we do together: it is a socially embodied medium of understanding and adjustment in which people engage in practices of allotting, assuming, or deflecting responsibilities of various kinds. These practices create a vocabulary, as it were, that lets us understand who must or may do something for or to someone, and they contain resources for moral deliberation that give us recognized and socially shared ways of deciding what is good or right to do. On this view morality is *expressive* of who we are, morally speaking, as well as of who we would like to become. And it's *collaborative* because it both presupposes and seeks a common moral life. This is not to say that the moral understandings that operate in a community are endorsed by all or that everyone understands the same things, but the members of the community do try to go on together—though not always fairly—negotiating in an ongoing process the moral terms that make a shared life possible (Walker 1998).

Because the process is ongoing, past understandings have to be revised to take into account new situations, and the revised understandings may need to be projected onto the future. Ongoing negotiation also means that if we want to figure out how best to resolve a moral conflict, we have to know where other members of the community are coming from, and how we all got into this mess in the first place. For all of this knowing, we need narratives: narratives that display who we are, narratives that depict the history and possible future of our relationships, and narratives that trace the shifts in our shared understandings. As I hope I've now shown, there are at least seven things we can do with these narratives we need. We can read them, invoke them, compare them, construct them, counter them, analyze them, and parody them. And we do these things with stories so routinely we rarely think about it. So now, think about it, and consider too what this narrative activity shows us about our actual practices of morality.[1]

## Notes

[1] Parts of this essay appeared in an earlier paper (2002), Narrative Ethics and Literature. In *The Handbook of the Philosophy of Medicine*, vol. 1, *Bioethics: A Philosophical Overview* ed. H. Tristram Engelhardt and George Khushf. Dordrecht: Kluwer.

# 5.
## *The paradoxes of pity*

Emmanuel Housset

Pity is in itself a paradox, since, on the one hand, it is a fundamental dimension of human existence and not a peculiarity of the mind that one might or might not possess. Indeed, a man devoid of pity would be equally devoid of his full humanity, simply because he would have lost his capacity of sensitivity (*sensibilité*). Without pity, man would have no other possibility except that of sensing (*sentir*) himself, and therefore there would be neither world nor neighbor nor community to affect him and to trouble the illusory tranquility of his self-presence. In truth, a man without pity would be equally pitiless towards himself; he would constantly be his own impartial judge, and it is easy to imagine why such an existence, which has all the appearances of wisdom, would in fact be hellish. Even so, on the other hand, experience teaches us that pity can be dangerous and irrational, and this is why in philosophy pity often has a bad name. One reproaches pity as a mere sentiment and therefore as hard to define and lacking in rationality. Sentiments are rarely objective and do not distinguish between good and evil. Good sentiments in general, and pity in particular, often lead to evil actions, and thus pity cannot exercise any moral authority. Philosophy denounces pity as extremely dangerous, because it pretends to make us act righteously while saving us the trouble of going through any reflection, any consultation of reason. Moreover, pity is uncontrollable and excessive: it can make us empathize with the worst criminal simply because a particular circumstance arouses our sympathy for him. Criminals can sometimes be so nice.

Conversely, pity can be absent for contingent reasons, simply because we are not moved by the misery of others. Our capacity to be pitiless, indifferent, is sometimes as astonishing as our capacity to burn with a bonfire of emotion, and one could be led to think that pity does not possess any faculty of discernment of its own.

## 1. The necessity of a concrete ethics.

Such is the paradox of pity: it is at the same time insufferable and indispensable, dangerous and a deliverance. Now, it is necessary to start from such a paradox if we do not want to limit ourselves to a formal ethics, to an abstract formulation of duty without reference to our engagement in and with the world, but rather want to develop a concrete ethics, one that starts from human experience itself. Indeed, pity leads to the questioning of ethics itself, because it forces us to ask where the "you must" is being formulated, that is: where respect for the other really originates, since pity can appear both as the foundation of this respect and as the form of its negation. In all its forms, pity is an extreme experience, because in it I can be closest to the other, but also most radically estranged from him, and it is from such an extreme experience that light can be shed on the nature of respect. Pity therefore is a privileged ethical phenomenon, and it is in trying to describe the phenomenon that it will be possible to understand when pity is good and when it is bad, since here good and bad are not predetermined values that would only need to be applied, but they are what needs to be clarified starting from any concrete situation of human existence. We should not allow ourselves to fall into the trap of a pure relativism that would lead us to deny the absolute value of the fundamental ethical law "thou shalt not kill," but nor is it possible to be satisfied with a formalism that does not try to determine what I must do for this person that I encounter. Indeed, pity speaks our humanity when it consists in an attention shown to the non-interchangeable singularity of the other, when it sees the other, not only as a particular example of the human species, but as an absolute singularity, as a unique history that does not compare with any other. Respect for man as my fellow, as sharing with me the dignity of being human, demands that reason be listened to, but it does not stand in need of compassion. Compassion is not necessary for the recognition of the other as a person, but it is indispensable for the encounter with another individual: without it, the other remains to me an idea, a function, a role, and he gives himself therefore as a general essence particularized by his place in the human world. Now, there is no compassion for man in general, not even for a character, but only for another flesh (*chair*), who in his unique sensitivity is at the same time close to me and yet always distant. True pity is a proximity that does not suppress the distance between two interiorities, because to be compassionate is not to take hold of the other as an *alter ego* but rather to hear what is unique and at the same time incommunicable in his suffering. From that point of view, if pity can be the source of respect, it is a kind of respect full of reverence (*pudeur*), of restraint, that tries to listen to the singularity of the other without reducing him to a "fellow man". That is the new paradox of pity: it is a communication in which the separation of interiorities, far from being suppressed, is on the contrary presupposed, since there is no truly human coexistence without a recognition of that alterity.

Here again one has to let oneself be taught by experience, to put between brackets such overhasty classifications as egoism and altruism, which most often are understood psychologically, that is, as a subject's dispositions. Such an interpretation conceals the fact that pity depends neither on me nor on the other, but can only be understood starting from the event of the encounter itself. The paradoxes of pity therefore point towards the necessity, but also towards the extreme difficulty, of not interpreting pity psychologically from the start, of not making it immediately into a product of the "I", because pity is, precisely, a modality of being in the world that precedes the possibility of saying "I". Indeed, pity is not first of all a voluntary act, not the product of a decision, but rather it invades me, it leaps on me, it is a modality of my exposedness to the other, who not only is a body in front of me, but who is a flesh (*chair*), a sensitivity starting from which I experience myself. It would seem, then, and this is not the least of the paradoxes, that pity is anterior to the distinction between "I" and "you" and therefore anterior to intersubjectivity. Compassion is an attitude whose source is not solely in myself, as shame is, but it is the way in which, in spite of myself, I am being thrown into the experience of the other and starting from which it becomes possible to establish the distinction between my lived experience and the other's lived experience. In this way pity puts me into question, makes a question of me, because I cannot know who I am except in my response to the possibilities that pity seems to indicate in me: it is starting from pity that I can understand myself as hardened or as sensitive. Therefore, pity makes a paradox of man himself to the degree that it forces him to no longer regard himself as a being endowed with conscience, to liberate himself from this abstraction of a closed interiority, of a "I" without a world wondering how to gain access to another "I".

Moral life cannot consist in conforming to an exterior model but consists in taking charge of the concrete situations in which our existence finds itself in order to ask ourselves what we have to do here and know. With pity as a first experience that opens the space of encounter and of dialogue, we have to discover moral norms that are not merely formal nor habits sedimented through the ages. Moral norms are living, that is, really operative, only when they are not mere habits and when they do not find themselves in some external or internal intellectual heaven, but when they are, in a way, received from the event of the encounter itself. Therefore, pity seems to make clear what "sensing" properly means: to be at the same time most intimately oneself and most outside of oneself. Every sentiment, and pity in an extreme way, is at the same time what is most interior and what is most exterior, and this is why it can make a duty possible. The duty to love one's neighbor cannot come from a purely reflexive experience, from the fact of being the pure spectator, first of oneself and afterwards of others, because one's neighbor is precisely not just an object of sight but is, on the contrary, that which seizes me in an immediate communication of a sensing (*un sentir*). Only a transcending lived experience can create a duty, because in calling me out of myself, such an experience places me in a situation in which I have to respond to the other prior to any rule concerning equality or reciprocity.

## 2. Dangerous pity

In order to understand the nature of pity, it is necessary to clarify this dangerous pity further, to use the title of a celebrated novel by Stefan Zweig, insofar as this dangerous pity does not allow for respect but is the expression of a form of contempt. This study is necessary on conceptual grounds, in order to distinguish between two totally opposite forms of pity, but it is also necessary on existential grounds, since nobody can with certainty distinguish clearly for himself between good pity and bad pity. From Seneca to Spinoza to Kierkegaard, philosophy has often described that so-called pity that is nothing other than the form of our egoism, but surely it is Nietzsche who has given its most systematic critique. The unrelenting critique of pity in Nietzsche is linked to the critique of the "I": our being overflows this so-called "I", because our conscience is too narrow to grasp what happens in us, notably our instincts. Thus, our isolation connected to the will to possess ourselves gives rise to the illusion that it is the I that produces thought, whereas it is rather thought that produces itself in me, to the degree that it is not just an intention of conscience but also a state of the body. To break with the illusion of a substantial I leads also to a break with traditional morality centered around an I and which, under the guise of disinterestedness, is a form of egoism. Hence the Nietzschean refusal of pity is not the Kantian refusal of all that is pathological in order to act out of sheer will, but is the refusal of the morality of the good man to which he opposes an ethics beyond good and evil, which he sometimes calls "immoralism" and which to Nietzsche does not mean outside of any law and any order. The radical, and it should be admitted more and more violent,[1] critique of compassion in the work of Nietzsche is a critique of Christianity understood as a popular idealism, and this is why Nietzsche places in opposition, sometimes a bit too easily, the love of the one nearby (*prochain*) and the love of the one far away (*lointain*).

In this critique of compassion, Nietzsche's aim is to denounce the reduction of the sentiments in general and love in particular to a purely subjective dimension, and for this reason he seeks to attack Christianity at its core, that is, to attack its definition of love. The strength of Nietzsche's analyses is certainly the refusal of a too simple opposition between egoism and altruism, of love of self and love of the other, which he wrongly attributes to Christianity, with the aim of re-evaluating the body and egoism, but without returning to an idealistic ethics.

Nietzsche is rightly cautious about a "pure" morality, which often masks an all-too-human morality: if compassion is a value, and even the value of Christianity, is this not the simple result of its utility? Isn't pity called good only because it is useful to us? Nietzsche wants to show that compassion is neither a good "in itself" nor an evil "in itself" but that it is bad when it weakens our power and good when it intensifies it. Put another way, in ethics it is necessary not to abstractly oppose good and evil: all disinterested action is always at the same time interested, and if one praises disinterestedness it is often out of interest. As a consequence, the critique of altruism is in no way a eulogy of egoism, but it is the concern to show the ambivalence of moral life: if a good inclination can reveal itself as bad, then a bad impulse can also participate in the quest for some good. Everyone has to come to realize at least once in his life that his compassion is not necessarily pure and that his insensitivity is not necessarily bad.

In paragraphs 132 to 136 of *Daybreak*, Nietzsche gives a systematic critique of the morality of pity of Schopenhauer and John Stuart Mill as "last echoes of Christianity in morals" (Nietzsche 1881, § 134). Indeed, Nietzsche's "unthinking man", who could be the man in the street just as well as the philosopher, believes that he acts purely out of compassion when he saves someone from drowning or when he relieves the pain of someone who is ill, but in fact he thinks only about himself. We often act either out of fear of shame (what would people have said of me had I done nothing?) or out of fear of our own fragility (I relieve this person of his pain because I cannot stand it), or else we act for the glory of playing the strong man, the savior (I am humanity's benefactor). Therefore we need to beware of those who want the good for us, because sometimes they want only their own good; and it is entirely reasonable to attack, as Nietzsche does, the possibility itself of com-passion (*Mit-leid*), since in fact there is no common suffering. One could argue that compassion aims only at liberating oneself from one's own suffering: one reacts to the suffering of others by an altruistic act in order to liberate oneself from one's own suffering connected to the wretched sight that the other gives us. Finally, in compassion it is the other that I do not think about, being preoccupied with myself: I enjoy myself in the act of helping the other, so that the other is only the occasion of my own satisfaction. Thus, in this bad compassion there is neither solidarity in suffering nor lucidity about the other: compassion blinds; moreover, it is suspected of being the will not to see. The praise of the unpitying man in *Daybreak* should be understood as a critique of a sentimental tenderness that is nothing else but another form of egoism.

Compassion can thus be understood as the greatest danger since it reveals itself as the contrary of what it pretends to be: it is an expression of contempt, of the will to diminish the worth and the will of the other; and so "benefactors" can be more dangerous than enemies, because they deprive us of the testing of our freedom itself, which occurs through enduring our suffering and our misfortune (Nietzsche 1882, § 338). Nietzsche denounces here all projects of a society kept on tranquilizers or painkillers: compassion would be the opium of the individual. From this point of view, according to him, the religion of pity finds its source in the religion of comfort, which avoids the test of suffering and tends to consider all suffering as bad. Because of this, Nietzsche opposes to the Christian ideal of the compassionate man the ideal of the doctor: "But he who, one way or another, wants to serve humanity as a doctor will have to be very wary of this sentiment (compassion),—it paralyzes him regularly at the decisive moment and annihilates his knowledge and his skillful, helpful hand" (Nietzsche 1881, § 134). The doctor is here the model of the noble man, who not only does not want to humiliate, but who also really wants to act in order to relieve suffering. The compassionate man, by contrast, in a way enjoys the suffering of the other, because in it he finds the source of his own power. In this devaluation of pity, Nietzsche will go so far as to say that compassion is a hatred of man, writing in §7 of the *Antichrist* that "pity is the practice of nihilism": it is dangerous for both the species and the individual, who either descends into melancholy or creates his happiness by affirming his superiority.

Against this dangerous, nihilistic pity, against this emotional sympathy that has crept into us through the centuries to the point that it has become a second nature, Nietzsche considers the possibility of another kind of pity, a pity of the strong. Whereas traditional pity is linked to our weakness and to our cowardice, the pity of the strong man, of whom the doctor is once again the model, would be a pity without pathos (Nietzsche 1881, § 142). While Nietzsche describes Christian pity as lacking in restraint (*pudeur*) and as limited to the neighbor, "our pity," says Nietzsche, "is a superior pity that sees further" (Nietzsche 1886 § 225). He adds in another text: "I like a pity that hides behind a hard shell: I like a pity in the name of which one breaks one's tooth".[2] Again, he writes: "I love the man who is so compassionate that he makes his hardness into his virtue and his divinity".[3] This hardness is no insensitivity but is what in *Thus Spoke Zarathustra* he calls discretion (*pudeur*), i.e. that restraint that opens us up to alterity, while compassion closes us up in ourselves.[4] True love for Nietzsche is the love that leads us to see the other as distant, i.e. without comparing the other to oneself, without making oneself the norm of what the other is: the thing is to love the "superman" in the other, which means that which he can become over and above all sentimentalism. Love does not melt together, it lives, rather, from distance, which is why Nietzsche sets up an opposition between the pathos of distance and the pathos of pity. Put differently, this discretion (*pudeur*) is what enables us to no longer consider the other from the point of view of our utility; it is that nobility which makes possible a true generosity and a true lucidity. My duty, that which I must do, comes not from God, not from the moral law within me, but from this experience of distance. In a way that became more and more violent, Nietzsche dedicated himself to the destruction of the *caritas* that is the enemy of life: "Compassion, *caritas*, while making it possible for the oppressed, the weak to survive and to have a posterity, contradicts the natural laws of evolution: it accelerates decay, it destroys the species,—it *negates* life".[5] Against the Christian love of compassion, which is a love of the weak for the weak, Nietzsche opposes the love of the superman, the man beyond nihilism who can love beyond compassion.

It is impossible to make an in depth study here of the fundamental concepts of Nietzsche's thought, but it is sufficient for our study of compassion to underline that, although Nietzsche sees in compassion the very expression of nihilism, although he relentlessly denounces in it a "yes" to the other which is in fact a "no" to the other, it is nevertheless the case that he is content with this generalized denunciation of *caritas* without really explaining the nature of the true "yes" to the other. As a result, if Nietzsche's analyses effectively free us of a dangerous pity that in reality is only self-enjoyment and contempt of the other, which is nothing but a feminine fear of suffering and not a will to elevate oneself above suffering, it has to be admitted that Nietzsche does not elucidate the character of the pity of the strong, that pity without pathos. Certainly, in *Human, All Too Human*, he overthrows pity in order to commend cordiality, affability, and kindness of heart, but that is a rather meager result that leads to this contradiction of a pity that does not suffer (Nietzsche 1878, § 49).

We return here to the core of the paradox of compassion: Nietzsche cannot really endorse another form of pity, and thus another form of love, since his criticism is aimed at the very essence of pity, and one wonders how a man without pity could be a sensitive man. In destroying Christian *caritas* as all too human, he also destroys all possibility of love and is left with an abstraction, this time not human enough, of a love that would be nothing but the expression of force. Between the superman and the compassionate man no reconciliation is possible, and one has, in a way, to choose between two forms of understanding of love: should love be a pure expression of the will to power, or does it consist in being strong in one's weakness? Certainly,

Nietzsche has not understood the Pauline theme of force in weakness and has arbitrarily reduced *caritas* to weakness, but it remains nevertheless the case that in Christianity compassion is the very nature of love, because weakness can be a source of virtue, while for Nietzsche it is always an evil. Nietzsche notably praises cheerful passions in order to denounce pity as depressive, but that leads him to refuse any form of passivity and to build the dangerous abstraction of a passion that would only be active. As a result, if Nietzsche teaches us that true pity should not be a flight in the face of suffering, it remains for us to understand what it means to form ourselves starting from suffering, that is, what it means to be compassionate.

### 3. Compassion as an incarnated virtue.

The difficulty with a concrete ethics is to understand, in concord with what experience teaches us, that there is a truth inherent in emotions and sentiments and that it is impossible to push them aside completely, into the region of the irrational. Man is not a pure mind, and it is as a whole being, soul and body, that he can experience compassion when he turns towards the other, not in order to use this other, but in order to let him manifest himself, to accompany him in his existence. Sensitivity belongs to our humanity, and we have already seen that a completely dispassionate man, devoid of all pity, would be an alien to us, stranger in a way than any animal. Nevertheless, in order to understand the significance of this sensitivity it is necessary to go beyond the opposition between the love of the one nearby (*prochain*) and the love of the one far away (*lointain*), which does not allow us to explain the self-forgetfulness that is part of compassion. Indeed, in true compassion, it is not I who forget myself, even in an illusory way, but it is the other who pulls me out of myself and gives a possible sense to my life. Life is going beyond oneself, but this does not consist in going beyond oneself in order to fulfill one's role, be it that of educator, of political leader, or of doctor. In such an idea of "self-effacement",[6] becoming oneself is still understood in terms of sheer will, while compassion cannot be understood as based solely on the will, since it is not something that one creates in oneself, even unconsciously. Pity is a sentiment received from the encounter with the other, and, like suffering owing to love, it is not at first a voluntary suffering, even if it can become so afterwards: in it, the power to exist and to act come precisely from the distant one (*lointain*), and this is why in pity one is taken beyond oneself. Consequently, compassion is never that disinterested love of humanity in general, nor the love of the superman: its aim is not to love an impersonal essence or what man could become beyond his weaknesses, but to love the concrete individual person as he gives himself, with his unique history and flesh (*chair*). The other in front of me is not one more copy of the human kind, nor an individual who has to learn to hide behind his role, but he is that unique being who sends me out of myself and into exile, because he asks something of me, because he calls upon my knowledge or at least upon my presence. Nietzsche may celebrate the courage of the act of losing oneself and perishing in order to become a new man,[7] but this harder attitude of wanting eternal steadfastness is still another form of pride, and this is completely contrary to compassion, in which it is the unimaginable and gratuitous character of the encounter that makes a new man of me, since it develops in me possibilities that I could not imagine possessing and that I could not have given myself by myself alone. Thus one sees that it is impossible to separate sensitivity and duty, insofar as sensitivity is not first a movement of closing myself in within myself, but should be understood as an openness without which there would by neither world nor neighbor.

This re-evaluation of pity, the understanding of weakness included, aims to show that our body participates in our being-in-the-world, and Thomas Aquinas already pointed out that the body is not a burden to overcome but is indispensable if the soul is to fulfill its essence. To become a man therefore not only consists in developing one's mind, but is also a task of incarnation, since man is a body that becomes intelligent. Concretely, one develops one's humanity by putting to work one's rational capacities, in Plato's phrase, by becoming a pure glance towards the intelligible, but also by learning to become present in person *en chair et en os*—"in flesh and bones," as the French expression goes—to the world. Experience shows that the human body is not primarily the place where self-consciousness occurs but is first of all the place of a receptivity, of a listening to things, to one's neighbor, and even to truth. Certainly, the body (*corpus*) is also flesh, and *caro* reveals here the fragility of sensitive man, nevertheless since Tertullian this fragility is also regarded as the possibility of salvation. Indeed, from Tertullian to Thomas Aquinas, flesh (*caro*) has been understood not as being in itself bad but as the place where our humanity puts itself in balance: either I become hardened and inward-looking or I turn myself towards the other. Indeed, for Thomas Aquinas, as for a good many of the mediaeval philosophers, man cannot find his unity except by opening up to what is not him, and this is why he is by essence sensitive: he has to learn how to sense (*sentir*). Therefore, the passions—by which term Thomas Aquinas designates all movements of the sensible desire (*désir sensible*) and not just movements contrary to reason—really are the place of our humanity.

One sees that the importance of mediaeval ethics for us today is that it is thoroughly concrete and frees us from contemporary formalism by describing the situations in which man finds himself entangled. There is, for instance, an anger which is not a vice opposed to softness but which is an expression of love. Thus, passions can be virtuous: "Yet it is true, as Saint Augustine has proven, that a certain form of sadness is praiseworthy when it procedes from a sacred love".[8] Returning more particularly to compassion, it shows that sensibility can be a place of strength and is not the danger denounced by Nietzsche; nor is it the substitute for virtue or the simple aid to virtue that it has often been reduced to. Far from being an *Ersatz* (substitute) for those who are not fully possessors of human wisdom, compassion can in itself be virtuous, when one considers it as an attention to others which is not judgmental, which does not make one singularity the norm of another singularity. Moreover, for Thomas Aquinas, compassion understood as *misericord* is at the same time a passion and a virtue, and that is why it can assure the unity of amorous passion and charity as a virtue. Indeed, charity is not a purely rational love, free of any pathological element, as Kant wished it to be, but is on the contrary a passion that has become virtuous without ceasing to be a passion. Duty is not what imposes itself on me in a bifurcation of conscience; it is on the contrary accomplished starting from an existence in the flesh in which it might perhaps never experience the other person's suffering directly, but I suffer because of his suffering. In a certain way, I can perhaps better commiserate with the other persons' suffering when I have not felt a comparable suffering myself, because in that case my sensitivity is more open. This confirms that an ethics without compassion would be a disincarnate ethics[9] where knowledge of what to do would not need to start from the experience of the other man. True compassion is not the hypocritical egoism described above, because it is this received capacity to become more sensitive and more lucid when faced with injustice or suffering. So there really is an intelligence of compassion in which my body is engaged to the degree that it is the condition of the perception of an evil and the condition of a questioning about its duty. Hence, there is no effective duty without such a bodily proximity that makes me into a question: Who am I in the face of this suffering? Am I the one who is going to consent to the desire to escape as far as possible into an existence of voluntary distraction, or am I the one who is going to make the effort to listen and accompany the other with the patience of love? Because this "Who are you?" does not come from me but from the encounter, it shows that only an affective duty is an effective duty, and that a duty without compassion, out of indifference for its object, would remain formal, without force, without ardor. Put differently, without compassion duty is only an external conformity, and beyond the critique of despising pity it is also necessary to critique the project of a pity of the strong that would be nothing but a form of hardening that would avoid all passivity, because it would be nothing but the project of a sensitivity without exposedness, without the risk of nakedness.

Nietzsche's relentless critique of Christianity in general and of pity in particular has made it impossible for him to see that Christian philosophy fought, long before he did, the abstract ideal of a life without affects, and it has, this time unlike him, recognized in pity the truth of affect without reducing the diversity and multiplicity of affects. Thus, life cannot be just an aspiration to power in the multiplicity of affects, but it does not become properly human except for the aspiration to give that finds its origin in a thankfulness towards the other for simply being there. Compassion itself is not solitary in that as it has originated from an encounter; and yet compassion shows the essence of passion, because it shows how passion can be a virtue without being a passion, that is to say, a weakness. Compassion therefore cannot be understood if one starts from the alternative of power and weakness: if, as Thomas Aquinas demonstrates, there is only virtue when reason penetrates into the very intimacy of sensitivity, in this virtuous passion the force of reason presupposes sensitivity as weakness, as the capacity to be touched by the misery of others. Now, it is exactly sensitivity as weakness which makes me capable either of running away into an ontological and ethical egoism or of approaching the one who touches me by allowing his suffering to become my suffering, not in the sense that I would experience his suffering but in the sense that it would become what most preoccupies me. There is here the possibility of a true respect that knows how to reconcile intelligence and sensitivity.

Compassion can thus be understood as an expression of human wisdom, insofar as this suffering through love is a humility allowing us in its weakness and its finitude to respond to the other. In this respect, one understands better that an ethics based purely in the will to be oneself and to expand one's power cannot leave a place for compassion, because compassion demands a suspension, at least momentarily, of this self-affirmation, it demands that one limit oneself to assuming for eternity one's choices against dispersion. Certainly, it it not a question of submitting one's actions to the will of the other by renouncing one's liberty, without which there is no ethical life, but one also has to be wary of that hardening that consists of wanting absolutely what one wants, against everything and everyone. From this point of view, compassion is not really a value; it is rather what enables values to lose their rigidity in order to rediscover a suppleness that is necessary to action: compassion is not justice, but a justice without compassion can become unjust, because it is not attentive to individuals. To tell the truth is an absolute duty, but to tell it without compassion, that is, without attention to the one to whom we tell it and to his capacity to hear it, becomes a form of violence. Reason formulates the imperative to speak the truth, since to hide it is a form of contempt, but compassion, on the other hand, requires that we reflect on how to speak it so that it can be heard.

Man is not the Hercules that modernity sometimes dreams about, that is, a being capable of creating itself, perfectly in control of itself, without weaknesses, dedicated to the infinite task of accomplishing its essence and capable of enduring anything. If it is by our weakness that we are receptive to the other, then compassion as weakness of love cannot be infinite and no man is capable of taking upon himself all the suffering in the world. Such a recognition of the finitude of human compassion is indispensable, because it assures the possibility itself of compassion: if I can never be as compassionate as is necessary, I am at least assured that all finite acts of compassion are a good, and this certainty is what keeps me from losing myself in a feeling of impotence. This shows as well that compassion is not solitary, that it does not solely lock one into the relation between two persons, and that it presupposes a human community within which we learn to sense, to become available. Just as there is no man without body, there is no man without community, and it is together that we can learn respect for the other, it is in a community that we learn to be the guardian of the other and not his master, his judge, or his tutor. Between the dangerous pity described by Stephan Zweig and the pitiless pity of which the doctor would be the model according to Nietzsche, it is no doubt necessary to imagine a third way: knowing that I am not the judge of the other, knowing that in my weakness and in my finitude I cannot bear everything, knowing that one does not become oneself in solitude, I can understand that I am a witness belonging to a chain of witnesses and that compassion is this capacity to be witness and not spectator. The witness is thus the one who allows himself to be transformed by the other, the one who receives him starting from his fragility and his finitude and who turns this fragility into a force of presence and action. One understands then that if compassion is so badly thought of, even when it is not hypocritical and contemptuous, that is because it costs us so much, because it is in no way easy, because it demands that we renounce our "dear me" and our dream of all-powerfulness.

To conclude, it is possible to bring together the different faces of compassion by underlining that it is the source of true respect because it is fundamentally a patience, but a patience which is not a form of hardening, which is not a capacity to endure everything because it has become untouchable. One has to recognize then that compassion is the negation of nihilism because it frees us from an existence closed to others and centered around the persistence of the I. Compassion can also be understood as the bracketing of the sole care of oneself that makes possible a life of care for what is present before us and to what we have to respond. Thus the experience of compassion as the experience of an exile teaches us that in respect, my being is not where I am, but there where I have to do something in response to the appeal of the other. Compassion is then a commitment in patience by which I give the other the time to speak himself in order to better understand him, and in this it makes possible a community which is not a natural community, nor a community of self-interest, but which is that proximity in which I enjoy and suffer through, because of, another man. The decisive paradox of pity is thus that it is a sentiment that does not lock us up in ourselves but that, on the contrary, leads us to exist beyond ourselves by widening our sensitivity to that distance (*lointain*) that is the other, and this prior to any decision.

(Translation John Steffen)

## Notes

[1] The development of this violence in the critique of compassion follows the growing understanding of the will to power as the essence of being. See Nietzsche 1886, § 36. If the will to power is the original form of sentiment (*l'affect*) and the

truth of all sentiment (*l'affect*), compassion can only be a negation of life. Nietzsche holds on to the opposition between understanding life as a deployment of forces and the definition of life as weakness and abandonment. Of course, it remains to be seen whether Christianity lets itself get caught in this opposition or whether it is rather the refusal of such a simplistic opposition by attributing a force to weakness and in a way also a weakness in the pure will to power.

[2] *Posthumous Fragments* November 1882 – February 1883, nr. 91.

[3] *Ibidem*, 5 (17). See also 4 (114) and 5 (1).

[4] See *Posthumous Fragments*, 187, 10 (119).

[5] *Posthumous Fragments*, 1887-1888, 11 (361).

[6] Nietzsche, *Posthumous Fragments*, 1881, 12 (93).

[7] See *Posthumous Fragments*, 1882-1883, 4 (44).

[8] Thomas Aquinas, *Summa Theologiae* III, Question 46, art. 6.

[9] This supposes, of course, that the body not be seen only as an organized plurality of forces and thus understood on the basis of will alone in all its complexity, and that the human body be seen as inseparable from a "corps à corps", an encounter between bodies, and that this is not only a more complex organism.

# 6.

# *Ethics of care, asymmetry, recognition, pity and self-management*

Mieke Grypdonck

Asymmetry in caregiving relations is the theme of this book, and it addresses the contribution of recognition and pity in response to the asymmetry. In this contribution we will examine recognition and pity in relation to nursing care for persons suffering from a chronic disease.

## 1. Asymmetry and the ethics of care

The ethics of care emphasizes that the need for care is universal and not restricted to the sick, the handicapped, the incapacitated, or the disadvantaged. Needing and giving care are universal phenomena and members of society, in general, both need and give care (Tronto 1993). Care giving and care receiving are often reciprocal, as is usually the case in family relations, but they also can be separated: the person from whom one receives care is not the same person as the one to whom one gives care. Nurses give care to patients, but also receive care—often from their patients or patients' family members, as our observations and interviews show. For example, patients are careful not to burden nurses unnecessarily. When a person recently having suffered a CVA was asked whether he talked to the nurses about it when he felt down, he replied that he didn't. "It makes the nurses feel bad", he said (Bouquez 1997). Nurses also receive care from their head nurse, from their spouse, from their friends. The ethics of care makes it clear, and it is certainly correct: the world is not divided into subjects who care and subjects who receive care.

Everybody is called upon to be both care receiver and care giver. Giving and receiving care is fundamentally human.

Although care giving and care receiving are both fundamentally human, many care situations are characterized by asymmetry: in caring for a family member, as exemplified in Kittay's report of her caring for her severely mentally handicapped daughter (Kittay 2003), in social care for the poor, in interactions in health care. Although both patients and nurses need care, and both are dependent upon this care, their situation is not similar, and there is a serious power imbalance (van Heijst 2005). While the nurses can either mentally or physically forsake care or go away to get it elsewhere, patients often do not have this power. They are dependent on care and on the willingness of others to give them care in an appropriate way, in a way that really helps them. They cannot do without it. And if the care is not appropriate, or even offensive, they have to tolerate it: at best with the freedom only to take a mental position vis à vis their fate (compare Frankl 1963). The asymmetries in care situations contrast with the egalitarian ethos of modern democratic societies. A person's dignity and worth is measured in terms of her or his being equal to others, i.e. independent, free and autonomous.

Asymmetries in (health) care are due to a large extent to defects in the care arrangements or in the way they are executed, and should be remedied or corrected. However, to some, often significant extent, they are also unavoidable.

## 2. Pity and recognition in the nursing care of persons suffering from a chronic illness

In what follows I will reflect on two concepts central to this volume —pity and recognition—and their significance for the field that I have been involved in as a nurse-researcher: trying to contribute to the improvement of practice by studying the lived experience of persons suffering from a chronic disease. In particular I will look at the significance of these concepts in the field of what has come to be called self-management.

## *Self-management in chronic illness*

In medical circles and in some nursing literature and practices self-management is considered to be synonymous with adherence (Grypdonck 2005; Shortridge-Baggett 2002). The patient has certain rules to follow, either in taking medications or in life style measures. His disease requires it, and doctors should discuss and deliberate with patients how the treatment can best be given in order to fit as well as possible into the patient's lifestyle and his goals in life. The patient can only be expected to adhere to treatments that are mutually agreed. Nurses can play a major role in instructing and helping patients adhere to this mutually agreed regimen. However, our research, as well as that of others, has shown that more is involved in self-management (Grypdonck 2005). We find that persons who have to live with a chronic illness continuously make decisions about how they will carry out their treatment and the rules of their life style in order to be able to raise the quality of their life above the disease. They, indeed, practice self-*management*. They manage their life continuously to find the best fit, not just once when they discuss their treatment regimen with their physician, but every day when they make decisions about what they will or will not do. Their self-management can be adequate or inadequate. We define self-management as adequate if it contributes to achieving the goals in life or in a particular situation the person with a chronic illness has set for him of herself, and inadequate when it leads to deviations from them. A person suffering from diabetes whose daughter is getting married and who wants to participate fully in the festivity, decides not to watch his diet closely, but ends up in the emergency room with a hyperglycaemia. He can be said to have practiced inadequate self-management.

Self-management regimens can be very demanding. Our research on what it means to continuously restrict fluids, as is required of persons on dialysis, makes it very clear what it means to them and requires of them (Dewettinck, Grypdonck & Dhondt 2001). It is almost beyond imagination for people who are able to live as they please. Our studies among people faced with poverty and its associated hardships also show how difficult it is to follow life style rules when, because of poverty, life has very little to offer (Duprez & Grypdonck 2002; Simmes & Grypdonck 1999). It seems unreasonable to expect of people coping with the hardships of life by living one day at a time, that they should make sacrifices in order to build a better future. Indeed, the future is kept out of sight and a better future is very difficult to imagine.

Those responsible for health care in governments or insurance companies, nowadays, are very interested in issues of adherence. Adherence to medication and life style regimens is a major factor in cost containment of health care. On the other hand, promoting adequate self-management proves to demand a considerable amount of resourcefulness and is by no means always successful. Almost as a matter of course, health care officials decide and declare that a patient has to take responsibility for his or her own health. The former minister of health in the Netherlands put forward the idea that persons who had not been adherent would be excluded from the national insurance they are normally entitled to for the treatment of those complications that one could reasonably assume would have been avoided by a proper life style regimen. Fortunately, the government changed hands before such an idea could be implemented.

What, then, can the concepts of recognition and pity contribute in the context of an ethics of care, when taking care of people who have to follow a restrictive life style regimen and find it very difficult to do so?

Those who agree with the minister of health of the Netherlands —and *non desunt qui*—can be said to lack both recognition and pity. The consequence is that they consider reasonable the idea that those who do not engage in proper health behavior should pay the bill themselves. Solidarity, of which the national insurance policy is an expression, should not go so far as to pay for the consequences of their lack of will power. If patients fail to make the proper sacrifices that their condition requires, they should bear the consequences themselves.

Our studies, however, show that the decision not to adhere to a required treatment regimen is often not a free choice, not in the full sense of the word, even if it is expressed as if it were—"if I have to die sooner because I am still smoking, then that's just the way it is. I don't mind. What's life if I have to give up smoking?" Such expressions often cover up the inability to act otherwise, which is felt but cannot be admitted to. The idea of killing oneself because of behavior one does not succeed in controlling properly is too offensive to an ego which is often already severely damaged (Grypdonck 2005).

### *Recognition and self-management*

Recognition is used and discussed by Axel Honneth and Estelle Ferrarese as a concept for political ethics. Baart, in his theory of presence (Baart 2001) uses the concept of recognition in the direct care relationship. It is the latter track that I will follow here (see also Baart, this volume).

Recognizing constitutes a relationship, a relationship that does not see the other only or mainly as the bearer of a task to be accomplished—either the task of making sure that they behave as their health requires or, worse, of making the other behave so that the doctor is satisfied with the result and the nurse is seen as a capable professional. Recognition means seeing the other as the person they really are, and accepting them as such: letting oneself be impressed by the veracious image of the other (Baart 2001). Recognizing a person means relating to them not in their role (e.g. as a dialysis patient) but as a person, with a life history, with desires and hopes and disappointments, who carries the weight of previously made mistakes, with power and strength, but also with weaknesses that bring them to a situation where they should not be and do not want to be. Recognizing a person means accepting them as they are, unconditionally; it means that change is not a precondition for relating to them or for doing one's best to achieve whatever would make the other person more fully a person, whatever would make his life (a bit) more complete.

People non-adherent to fluid restriction are often not "recognized". They are seen as weak, as sinners, as people who refuse to do what is necessary. They are considered as not listening, as acting improperly. They have been told what to do and they are expected to behave reasonably. And they do not. They are talked to, they are told off for not behaving according to the rules, that are, are they not, in their own interest. In some centers they are even punished by having to dialyse longer or by having to come in for an extra day (Waterschoot 2006).[1]

Recognizing a person with a chronic illness who is to be instructed and advised about a therapeutic regimen means, in the first place, connecting with the person (and thus getting to know them) as they are: a person with a personal and family life, with a life history in which the disease has appeared at a certain moment and has caused some—or a lot—of changes and turmoil. It means knowing them as someone with hopes for the future and desires for the present which —as is often the case—are not always fully compatible. It means getting to know them as a person who has achieved certain things and had to cope with disappointments, a person with a life of their own, often not made easy by the disease. Nurses, and even more so doctors, often see a person with a chronic illness as a patient; in their view, the illness comes first, and people with a chronic illness often accept that state of affairs. In a visit that seldom lasts longer than fifteen minutes, time needs to be used economically. In such consultations there is no possibility of learning to know the other, and thus they cannot be recognized.

Recognizing also means trying to understand what it means for the other to have to follow a life style and medication regimen that thwarts normal life by imposing limits that one has to accept, knowing that someone who is healthy can never fully understand what that means. Unlike the doctor who, in our study about life style adherence among people living on a very low income and suffering from diabetes, said to his patient that he understood that the patient was not able to follow the prescribed regimen. Neither would the doctor, if he had to (Logghe & Peeters 2006).

In our approach to supporting people who have to live on dialysis (Grypdonck, Weldam & Litjens 2003) we let the nurses start by allowing the person needing dialysis to tell the story of their life.

Even when the nurse has taken care of the person for a long time, the story the person tells proves to be very enlightening for the nurse. The nurse now better understands what an enormous space dialysis takes up in the person's life, and hears that the dialysis is often only one of the ordeals the person has to cope with. "When you listen to their complicated lives, the nurses say, you hardly dare to demand anything of them (in this case to refrain from drinking and stick to the fluid restriction)" (Weldam, Litjens & Grypdonck 2004). They now understand that imposing their rules and expecting that the patient is wise enough to do what he is told, is not appropriate. It does not fit the situation the person is in.

The narrative of the person who needs to be on dialysis and needs to restrict their fluid intake reveals the person as they are. The person (re)presents themselves in the narrative and the nurse listens; listens as much as possible without passing judgment. The nurse lets the person show them self, gives up any preconceived image of the patient, lets the person emerge as they want to be seen, and recognizes them as they construct the representation of them self. That the nurse recognizes the person who needs to live on dialysis means that things will never be the same as before. Their relationship is fundamentally altered.

Being able to allow oneself to be recognized as one is requires also a process on the part of the person with the chronic illness. It requires a certain degree of self-esteem, as well as trust, that the other will not take advantage of the vulnerability that becomes apparent when one is recognized as one is. To let oneself be recognized does not mean that the person who is ill will, or even could, or should, relate events and behavior as they actually take place. A mother who does not get out of bed in time to get the children to school can say that she truly loves her children and is prepared to do anything for them. Her representation of herself is true: such are, indeed, her intentions. This being prepared is her true self. Sometimes, or even often, she does not manage to follow through. But not because she does not care. Equally, someone who says that he really cares for his health must not be thought of as lying or as giving socially acceptable answers because he does not manage to keep to his fluid restrictions. The self that really wants to take care of himself is his true self, and his problem is that sometimes (or often, or most of the time) he is not successful.

Sometimes, people do not want to be recognized as they are. They do not want to recognize themselves as they are. We regularly find such persons among non-compliant patients. They have made a mess of their life, and they know it but cannot face it. They make themselves unapproachable. They present themselves in a way that is not in accordance with who they are or with who they would like to be. They hide behind a mask that makes their real self invisible, to others and to themselves. In such cases recognition is not appropriate. Recognizing who they really are would require analyzing them and the situation they are hiding behind the mask. It requires a therapeutic relationship to which they do not and cannot consent and, hence, nurses do not have a mandate to act. Perhaps then, pity is all that is left? The nurse can hope that the acceptance of the person as encountered may lead to enough self-acceptance to accept help. We noticed that pity motivates some nurses not to leave a patient alone, in spite of the fact that the patient frustrates them considerably. When a patient dies as a consequence of not restricting his fluids, they are (properly) mourned. Pity makes it possible not to reproach the ill person because of their behavior. The nurses are capable of attending their funeral as a last tribute.

### *Pity and persons with a chronic illness*

Acts of pity are rooted in the belief that every human being is worthy of compassion and care, whatever their situation and their attitude, even when these do not lead to any improvement in their situation. Housset (2003; see also this volume) and Leget (Leget 2004; Leget & Olthuis 2005) consider pity as a professional virtue of great importance to adequate care.

Pity has not been and is not popular in nursing. It is certainly not popular in the circles of the (Dutch) Patient Movement. People with a chronic illness do not like the idea of being approached with pity. To start with, the pity of others places them in a category apart form those who are normal neither in need of, nor evoking, pity. As has been pointed out repeatedly [see for example Oderwald (1994), Charmaz (1991)] being considered normal, not being set apart from those who are not ill or handicapped is an important issue for people with a chronic illness. In the second place, those with a chronic illness tend to deal with their illness with stoicism rather than by bringing their suffering to the fore (King, Carroll, Newton, & Dornan, 2002). Our studies lead us to believe that this attitude is not only fruitful in their relationship with others, but that it also has a positive impact on their own mood. People with a chronic illness avoid falling into a deep hole by telling themselves that they are strong, that they can cope, that it all is bearable. These thoughts often are a very effective way of cognitive coping. Health care workers feeling and—even worse—expressing pity greatly endanger these coping strategies. Finally, people with a chronic illness demand a discourse of rights. They have the right to proper health care, the right to (financial and personal) assistance in order to participate in society, the right to proper treatment of their health problems, the right to consideration when they (make the effort to) participate in "normal" social life. Pity seems to make these rights less obvious and, of course, as pity is an emotion (Housset), one cannot guarantee proper care based on an emotion which is, by its very nature, poorly controllable. It is thus not only understandable but also reasonable that patients are afraid of pity. Some even hate it.

Pity is an emotion which underlines or creates and even radicalizes asymmetry. Those who have a chronic illness and who only want to recognize asymmetry in their relation with care providers when it means that they are in control, will not be pleased with any (expression of) pity on the part of their health care workers. That will also be the case with the people discussed above who aren't respecting their fluid restrictions and do not want to be seen as they really are. It is very unlikely that they would be happy to be the object of their nurse's pity. What happens, then, when a nurse *feels* pity for a patient, but cannot allow it to be expressed because it would offend that person? And is justice done when the nurse, out of pity and as a tribute to the person attends their funeral while the patient did not want to be pitied?

Pity, on the other hand, is an important element in caring relations, not only as a motivator to do what is necessary and sometimes far from easy. Pity also fosters a humane relationship that fits the situation the patient (or his family members) are in. In the data from our qualitative interviews with patients and family members, we find many appreciative testimonials to the pity apparent in the interaction of the health care workers.

Good pity, according to Housset (2003), is an attention to others which is not judgmental and gives room fully—I would say, *as much as is possible*—to the otherness and the singularity of the other. Good pity is not self-referential as bad pity is. Good pity is an emotion that is evoked by the awareness of the suffering of the other, and the sorrow and the pain felt is not the sorrow and pain evoked by the idea that, one day, one could be in a similar position (Boleyn-Fitzgerald 2003). Good pity is not self-referential in the sense that the pain or sorrow the nurse herself feels is simply the motivation to act on behalf of the patient, as is the case in bad pity (Housset 2003; Boleyn-Fitzgerald 2003). Thus, good pity requires knowing the patient. Knowing the patient in their life history and understanding the complicatedness of their life and understanding the burden in which the situation places them, the nurse feels pity for them and understands why compliance to their therapeutic regimen requires too great an effort from the patient. The pity evoked by the insight into the patient's situation makes the nurse "more sensitive and more lucid when faced with injustice or suffering" (Housset, this volume). Patients will greatly benefit from this sensitivity which will allow the nurse better to tune in to the patient's real needs.

Pity, as an emotion or perhaps as a cultivated emotion, can help nurses not to turn their backs on patients they cannot help. It can also help them to give considerate and sincere care to a person who, for reasons that now become understandable, exhibits behavior which is different from what one should accept as a professional. Linda takes care of Mr Johnson. He suffers from diabetes and his body is covered with ulcers. He reminds Linda of the biblical figure of Job. Linda has to do his dressings. It is a procedure that takes forty-five minutes. During that procedure, Mr Johnson does not stop cursing. He yells at Linda, asks her whether she has actually been trained as a nurse as he would not think so from how she does the dressings. Linda remains calm and friendly. She says to Mr Johnson that she understands that the procedure is very painful for him, both literally and in the figurative sense. She will do her best to cause as little pain as possible. She will stop when he asks her to do so. And she knows, although she cannot fully understand, that he must suffer a great deal from his disease. Mr Johnson calms down a little bit, but only a little bit. The next day, Linda volunteers to take care of Mr Johnson. She knows she can cope with his curses, and thinks it is better for him to be able to curse than to be told that he has to respect his nurses or else they will refuse to carry out the procedure. She feels pity for Mr Johnson and that allows her to give him personal, sensitive and sincere care.

Pity does not preclude appreciation of the patient's (or family member's) strengths, as is sometimes suggested (Diggins 2007). This is apparent in the following case, taken from our interviews with parents of children that will die soon of cancer. The mother tells us how she reacted when her 10 year old son, whom she had just put to bed, and with whom she was lying in bed for a while, asked her, as they were speaking about the cancer in his head: "Do you think I will celebrate my 18$^{th}$ birthday?" The mother tells us

> He knew he had cancer, and he knew that he would die, but I had not told him yet how soon. It is so difficult to tell it all at once, so I said 'That you are asking that... I find it so very difficult to answer, because, you know, this is what makes us so terribly sad, and it is so hard to tell, because it is so hard for you to hear.' I said 'the doctors in the hospital have said ...' I have expressed it in months... 'maybe three, maybe two, may one month... So soon it can all be finished.' I said 'that is certainly very hard to hear.' (...) And, at the last moment, that is so terribly difficult for us as parents, yes, also for us as Christians, that you have to let him go... that he would not be anxious that he will be alone, so I said 'at the end, we will keep your hand, papa and I, and we will be with you... until Jesus comes and takes your hand, so you will not be alone, not one moment.'

> And for him, that was a great consolation, that he thought, that is the way it will happen. He was not afraid. (Kars c.s. 2009)

We cannot read this excerpt in our research group without feeling great pity for this mother, but at the same time expressing our admiration for the courage and the competence shown in this extremely difficult situation. And, as the mother teaches us, pity does not preclude proper and thoughtful action, even if what needs to be done will be painful, both for the giver and the receiver of care. The mother also shows us how and why pity is a virtue: something that is positive only if moderated by sensitivity and thoughtfulness.

## 3. Recognition, pity and asymmetry

Are recognition and pity (partial) answers to asymmetry in the nurse-patient relationship? They certainly do not redress the asymmetry, but we would contend, as our analysis has shown that they can be of great value in (highly) asymmetrical patient-caregiver relations. Many questions, however, remain. Perhaps answers would be easier to give if the value of concepts such as recognition and pity, but also of autonomy and asymmetry were more tailored to specific situations. In caregiving relationships it is often counterproductive to think in universals. What is appropriate and does justice to one type of person in one type of situation may be inappropriate or inapplicable in another situation. The ethics of care takes the specifics of the situation into account when judging how best to do right to an individual. The question should then be rephrased as: in what circumstances can recognition and pity contribute to the alleviation of uneasiness that follows from the asymmetry that is unavoidable in caregiving relations, given that the negatively perceived and avoidable asymmetry has first been corrected. It is certainly a question worthy of further investigation.

## Notes

[1] When patients have a fluid overload, dialysing longer or an extra time may be the best solution. However, it is presented to the patients as a punishment that is imposed by the doctors.

# 7.
# *Compassion in the context of an academic medical center*

Carlo Leget

In this contribution, we will reflect on the possible role of compassion in an ethics of care by relating Housset's analysis of compassion (*la pitié*) to the world of medicine and departing from our own work with medical students (Housset 2003). Our focus will be limited to one profession within health care, that of the physician, and our primary focus will be the role of compassion in their moral development. This allows us not only to speak of what we know best, but also to shift the reflection onto the question how we educate young people and prepare them to play a central role in the health care system of the future.

In this contribution we will move in two directions. We will outline some of the problems one meets teaching ethics to medical students and explain why we think Housset's analysis is worth taking to heart. Secondly, we will also propose four critical questions designed to help in performing a further analysis which will itself determine the proper place of compassion in an ethics of care.

In this contribution, education in medical ethics is considered not so much an intellectual mind game or a training in solution oriented ethical engineering, as an intellectual and emotional formation of the mind and the heart (Coulehan 2005). The minds and hearts of first year medical students are normally regarded as rich soil for moral education. Yet when you ask first year medical students why they have chosen to study medicine, they often express a desire to help people. This motivation can be considered as an important source for both the development of morality and for moral education. Yet, to our knowledge, it is hardly tapped in the medical curriculum.[1] Since being a physician is a demanding profession in relation to ethics and emotions, this is peculiar. Given that many medical students (and even physicians) consider medical ethics as an exercise that has little relevance to their professional work, one might even ask seriously how effective and successful the medical education of young doctors is at all (Bertolami 2004).[2]

## 1. Barriers in teaching ethics and Housset's contribution

In our experience, when teaching and discussing medical ethics with medical students one meets a number of barriers. Some of these barriers are related to the age of the students. Aristotle argues that good ethical deliberation requires a certain maturity, and the majority of medical students are bright, young and energetic, but far from mature. More fundamentally, however, there seem to be four widespread ideas that hamper ethical conversations before they have really begun. These ideas are tied to certain moral presuppositions of contemporary North Atlantic culture (Leget 2004).

The first widespread presupposition is the idea that ethics is a matter of personal feeling. As one of our undergraduates expressed it: "Like all ethical points of view, it is a matter of personal feeling and belief and not of scientific foundation." The problem of an emotivist viewpoint like this is that morality becomes a private matter without any political (in the philosophical sense) dimension. Those who hold this view withdraw themselves into their private universes, unwilling to acknowledge the influence of the culture surrounding them.

The second presupposition is held by students who think that some issues have no ethical dimension because they are already covered by legislation. "We live in a free country, and any person is entitled to think about ethical subjects as he or she believes, as long as the law is not violated", is what one often hears in discussions. The problem with this viewpoint is that it overlooks the interrelation of ethics and law. For example, in both the Netherlands and Belgium there is a clear relation between public morality and legislation concerning the last stages of life. For many students, however, it is a difficult task to understand the relation between personal convictions and the community.

A third problem is the widespread consequentialistic point of view by which the meaning and goodness of an act is limited to its consequences. This consequentialistic way of reasoning fits well in a problem solving mentality that is trained and fostered during medical school. In ethical discussions on end-of-life issues, e.g., many students find it hard to make a difference between putting an end to life (the physician inducing death) and taking care until the end of life (the disease inducing death). Although they admit that the distinction is vital in the legal difference between a natural and an unnatural death, in the end they think there is no moral difference, especially when a patient is severely suffering.

A fourth way in which the ethical conversation can be frustrated is when students say that their conviction is based on their religious belief. Religious convictions are respected among medical students in the Netherlands. However this respect reflects a negative concept of freedom that does not lead to a real conversation among students. Community is understood as a collection of individuals who do not bother one another and are free to believe what they want as long as they do not harm others. Moreover, many students, unfamiliar with religious traditions, think that religious perspectives are not open to reasonable debate.

This short sketch introduces some themes that are important for medical ethics education. Firstly, the relation between reason and emotion is important for young physicians who are confronted with events that move the emotions, and it raises the question to what extent emotions may have impact on moral decisions. Secondly, the idea of the community is relevant to the institutional context in which young physicians develop their professional attitude. Thirdly, the meaning of actions where they are related to the symbolic dimension of medical actions that students should be aware of. And finally the issue of respect is important regarding the basis of the relationship between physicians, other team members and patients.

Of these four issues, the idea that ethics is a matter of personal feeling is the most fundamental dogma. Successful education, we think, rejects the firm roots that particular dogma has in contemporary culture. It is precisely here that Housset's analysis can be helpful in confronting the problems that we discovered teaching medical ethics (Leget & Olthuis 2007).

In the first place, Housset shows that words are valuable and that inflation of words hampers the discussion of ethics. The word "respect" is easily used in discussions but it can have different meanings. The same goes for compassion. What we need in discussions is a permanent hermeneutics of these words. Such a hermeneutics is an exercise in simultaneously listening well and thinking precisely. No one asks of physicians that they should become philosophers. However, it belongs to their professional competence to be able to listen very attentively and carefully and to be aware of the multilayered content of words. Moreover, in order to understand the inner feelings of their patients and themselves they need a certain level of education and refinement in their thinking.

In the second place Housset's analysis shows that in its originary form compassion is not a degrading emotion. It can be a source of morality. Although it is acknowledged that ethics is a matter of one's own feeling and belief, one's self cannot be thought of as an isolated core of subjectivity. Real compassion is no self-affection but a coinciding of otherness and intimacy. There is a real connection with the world that enables morality. It is important to be aware of the fact that when one is touched by someone else's misery, the otherness inside oneself is revealed. The moment that one is struck by real compassion cannot be decided as an intentional act. Nevertheless, as with all emotions, one is touched in one's most subjective inner core. Of course there is always the possibility of cutting oneself off to feelings of compassion on the one hand, or enjoying self-affection of the other. Both options, however, are perversions of the originary experience.

All this means, in the third place, that compassion is the foundation of a form of community. In a pre-moral sense this is the case because—as we have seen—the originary experience of compassion reveals that I am connected with another person, even to the degree of accepting his pain and sorrow, before I even realize it. By consciously accepting the other person's misery—the moral act of compassion—the pre-moral sense of community is accepted. Subsequently one discovers a moral responsibility for the way this pre-moral community is fostered, threatened or denied by the institutional dimension of society. Because of that personal responsibility, as a physician one cannot hide behind the law or the institutional context of the hospital. There is always a moral choice in adopting a role, a position or a profession.

We think that the analysis of Housset is very helpful as a theoretical basis that helps in seeing firstly the importance of a continuous critical hermeneutics of the word "compassion"; secondly, the possibility of compassion as a source of morality and thirdly, the fact that compassion constitutes and reveals a form of community. But is that sufficient as a foundation for the education of young professionals?

## 2. Critical questions and further refinement

If we take compassion as a point of departure for the moral education of medical students, and if we accept Housset's analysis as a welcome contribution to this enterprise, we are still in need of further clarification. We will take four topics for further reflection, discussion and debate: the power and impact of the health care system; the problem of justice; and the place of negative emotions. As a last check we want to discuss the question whether compassion is really needed or whether it is better to confine oneself to the concept of empathy.

### *The power and impact of the health care institution*

Although one of the really strong points of Housset's analysis is that although compassion is tied to concrete physical persons, his analysis can also be characterized by some "disincarnatedness" in the fact that his subject is an abstract moral subject. The subject he describes is Everyman, dissociated from a concrete context. But it is precisely this social context which is of great importance for the development of moral subjects. A social context consists of more than just the interpersonal relations between parents and children, teachers and pupils of peers. The French Philosopher Paul Ricoeur has worked out the importance of not forgetting the role of the institutions in the development of personal and moral identity, besides the importance of the self-narrative and interpersonal relations (Ricoeur 1992). Ricoeur's analysis can be complemented by the work of the French sociologist François Dubet who has shown how the institutional contexts themselves are not uniform, but composed of different logics that compete and result in systemic pressure felt by both health care workers and patients (Dubet 2002).[3] What does this mean for compassion as a basis for moral reflection and action?

In the first place, it is a well documented fact that the systemic powers inside health care institutions have a huge impact on the formation of moral character. Literature speaks of the "informal" or "hidden curriculum" in medicine consisting of the impact of role models in the period of internships, the influence of which is far greater than the official curriculum (Bloom 1989; Hafferty and Franks 1994; Hunnert c.s. 1996). One of the better titles one comes across while studying the moral development of medical students is: "The Natural History of Cynicism in Phycisians" (Testerman 1996). The study concludes that cynicism among medical students results from the struggle and balance that medical students experience as part of the professional socialization process (Collier 2002).[4] Important factors affecting their professional development include working under high pressure, having overloaded schedules, having a great deal of responsibility and too little time to get things done. Although written ten years ago, times have not changed and discussions nowadays concern whether it can be justified to reduce the duty week from 120 to 80 hours (Friedlaender 2006; Mittal and Portnier 2006).

Health care has become an industry, sometimes even booming business. People are making big money, planning careers, delivering all kinds of output. Even if individuals feel sympathetic towards the idea of re-instating compassion, it will largely remain dependent on the power and success of this particular individual as to what sense that re-instatement would make. This power can be formal (head of a department) or personal (role model), but that does not bring compassion to an institutional level—even taking into account that many health care workers are indeed struggling with compassion fatigue (Huggard 2003).

What's more, there may even be strong reasons for avoiding compassion, reasons that show a certain wisdom reaped from harsh experience. One is confronted with one's huge vulnerability and impotence in dealing with the patient's misery, with one's own dependency on an often inadequate and unfair system of health care, with the impossibility of running away and with one's own fragile existence.

Must we conclude then that there is no place for compassion in medicine? Despite the picture we have sketched, even the more prestigious medical journals can surprise. In 1999 the *Journal of Clinical Oncology* published a paper "Can 40 Seconds of Compassion Reduce Patient Anxiety?" (Fogerty 1999). We realize that a title like this may almost sound like a joke, a curse or an insult. Thinking back to the helpful analysis of Housset which we discussed earlier, it is obvious that there is a huge distance between the disruptive, patient-, and mystery-oriented analysis of compassion that he undertakes on the one hand, and the hasty, formal, result-oriented and problem-solving world of medicine on the other. Many articles on subjects such as compassion or spirituality in medicine have a similar status: they are tolerated, but only if (a) it is empirically documented that they have a positive result, (b) they are instrumental and (c) do not take too much time (Sulmasy 2006).[5] On other words: they are tolerated as long as they do not interfere with the real business of medicine.

And yet, from time to time there is also a different voice to be heard. The prestigious *Journal of the American Medical Association*, for instance, has the good tradition of reserving some pages that are addressed to the inner self of the physician: "A piece of my mind", these pages are called, and sometimes these minds are the minds of beautiful people. One of these short contributions is titled "The subtle power of compassion" and tells the story of a doctor who is impressed by what a former patient of her tells. In her own words:

> The power of compassion is subtle. It may never be acknowledged by the recipient. It may never be rewarded by a promotion or a public recognition. Sometimes it comes across in a few words or a smile or a kind glance or a few extra minutes of time. Yet its effect can last a lifetime.

Apart from the fact that, again, the measure of time plays a role here, we hear a different voice. A voice that is more consonant with the phenomenological analysis of Housset. These voices, however, are small flowers in a huge desert, and cannot bring the concept of compassion to an institutional level. If we really want to reflect on compassion as a promising concept, we will have to understand better what factors make it so hard to keep these small flowers alive; we will have to understand better what health care institutions do with people, and how on an institutional level, compassion can be fostered. That means that we will have to gain more insight into the way the different logics inside institutions create tensions and oppositions. One of these logics is related to justice. That brings us to our second point.

### *The problem of justice*

The disruptive experience of compassion, so well analysed and described by Housset, has important heuristic and formative possibilities. As such it seems that it should be part of the emotional formation of all those who work in health care. There is, however, a much debated problem with compassion: the fact that its disruptive force brings about a strong impetus to focus on one single patient or event. How is this related to the ethics of care perspective?

If we take it as characteristic of the ethics of care that in order to find out what is good for the patient it pays attention to (a) the unicity of specific situations, (b) the asymmetry that is given with dependency, (c) the vulnerability linked to our bodily existence and (d) the importance of being–in–relation, then at first sight, compassion seems to impose itself as the royal road (van Heijst 2006). By compassion one is drawn into being–in–relation: compassion is inflamed by the perception of someone else's vulnerability, and this is done so strongly that the unicity and specificity of the situation prevails. Whether compassion is related to asymmetry, and whether it implicitly degrades someone else is disputed, as Housset has shown. But he has also demonstrated that there is a way of understanding compassion in which the asymmetry is acknowledged without any degradation. Nevertheless, there is still one big problem that comes into sight when we realize that every care relation is embedded in the larger web of the people we are related to. By touching the heart of the caregiver, the pre-moral experience of compassion highlights unicity and risks arbitrariness and injustice from the perspective of other vulnerable people. Notably those who are so unlucky that nobody feels anything for them (Batson 1995). All these problems raise the question whether we do indeed need a second, independent source of moral discernment as well as the more emotional one of compassion.

One of the wise proposals of Paul Ricoeur in *Oneself as another* is to correct the primordial Aristotelian emotion and virtue-based intention of ethics ("aiming at the good life, with and for others...") with the more Kantian approach of "duty" ("... in just institutions"). This proposal is based on the idea that morality needs the filter, or even moral sources of deontology precisely because of our moral finitude. A more formal approach to good care in terms of justice can be linked to the previous point we made about the importance of taking into account the impact of the health care institution. It can be a source for rethinking the role of institutions in terms of justice. Perhaps compassion can only play a sound and solid role in an ethics of care if the care is provided only within institutions that guarantee a just and well– balanced compassion. In this sense "institutionalized compassion" might be as important for good care as the personal compassion of care givers, relatives or people passing by.

Despite this balance, however, one can still ask if we are thinking about the role of compassion on too narrow a basis of only positive emotions and intentions. This brings us to our third point of attention and discussion.

### *The place of negative emotions*

People who care for other people are confronted with different kinds of emotions.[6] Care is not always inspired by compassion: it can be related to a number of positive and negative feelings, emotions and motives. Let us begin by looking at two vignettes, based on real life events, to make my point a little more concrete. The first one concerns an unexpected event in the street, experienced by a citizen. The second one is told by an experienced medical professional.

> One summer evening I was walking to the train station, when suddenly a young kid (he must have been 18 years or so) fell off his bike. His head touched the ground and he did not move. My first reaction was one of irritation. I had seen him riding on the pavement, wobbling on his bike, and looking dopey. My instant impression was that he had taken pills or so. My instant reaction seeing him lying there was annoyance that I would miss my train. Nevertheless I felt I had to do something, so I picked my phone and started calling an emergency number. I did not leave until the ambulance had arrived. Looking back on the event I do not feel proud. In fact I do not feel anything at all. I am not even interested on how the kid is doing now. I would not call my reaction compassionate; it was just something I felt I had to do.

Let us take one step further and look at a second vignette.

> As a physician from time to time one has to deal with patients that arouse a certain disgust or even the feeling that they do not "deserve" to be helped. You may strongly dislike a person whom you have got to help. At this moment I have a patient that I find strongly unsympathetic and I don't think I feel any sort of compassion. I do know, however, that I have helped him in a decisive way and I am interested in him in a way. I do not think that I am not a good doctor because I do not feel compassion all the time. I think a good doctor is an experienced physician who knows what decency and good practice are, and who is able to "produce" these two even under difficult circumstances.

What do these two vignettes tell us about compassion? In the first place, they show two examples of situations where compassion, in the sense Housset describes it, is totally absent. In the first vignette there is no experience of any feeling at all; in the second one, the opposite of compassion is felt: a certain dislike or even disgust. Nevertheless, both situations can be considered as examples of compassionate action. Would it be wise now to add a third type of compassion, in addition to Housset's pre-moral experience of compassion and his moral (virtuous) version, compassionate behaviour?

Would it be wise to consider compassionate behaviour as an important professional quality? Is it really necessary—from the perspective of an ethics of care—to be emotionally involved, or can one simply do with compassionate behaviour? The obvious risk is that care is reduced and stripped to external and visible action and behaviour, neglecting the more relational, emotional and motivational elements involved. The good thing about compassion as behaviour, however, is that in the end care is more than just good intentions. Good care is measured by action. And taking compassionate action seriously, one is both realistic and pragmatic. In the end, caring is something that needs to be done. Of course it is to be preferred when care relations are sustained by emotions of sympathy and compassion, but let us not be too romantic about this.

Apart from the suggestion of focusing on concrete and external results in terms of caring behaviour, the two vignettes can lead us to a second insight, this time focusing more on the emotions that are related to the motivation of those who care. Would it not be important to complement Housset's phenomenological analysis of compassion with a phenomenological analysis of disgust, an experience that also touches our inner core and reveals "otherness"? Cultural anthropologists have shown, and Martha Nussbaum has worked out, how disgust propels demarcation and exclusion of moral communities (Nussbaum 2001, 2004). Instead of condemning it, one can also see the spontaneous experience of disgust as having important pre-moral content that tells us something about ourselves as moral beings. Perhaps an analysis of disgust in medical practice could be helpful in discovering one's boundaries as a moral subject. All medical students wrestle with these boundaries in other respects too: in their first anatomy courses, and in their relationships with patients, but equally in their professional life as well–trained surgeons (Dinsmore 2001). Focusing on disgust might be helpful in order to acknowledge the finitude and fragility of ourselves as moral beings.

Focusing on compassion can reveal important insights, but as we have seen, one might argue that it is better to take into consideration that there are sometimes negative emotions, or no feelings at all, but that these result nevertheless in compassionate behaviour. My suggestion is that, in order to be more concrete and realistic, we complement Housset's analysis with both recognition of compassionate behaviour and with research into the nature of negative emotions. But if we have that intention, why not forget about compassion at all, lower our standard and let empathy do the job?

### *Can empathy do the job?*

Reflecting on the role of compassion in health care, and taking the medical journals into consideration, one might be tempted to play all one's cards on a different but related concept: empathy. Much work on this concept has already been done, and it seems to have a relatively firm and steady basis in health care, being acknowledged as an important precondition for a good physician-patient relationship.[7] The development of empathy in medical students is identified as a key goal by the American Association of Medical Colleges (Medical School Objectives Writing Group 1999). And according to many medical journals it can be trained, measured and promoted (Mangione 2002; Benbassat & Baumal 2004). So why not take this less problematic and more clinically accepted concept and dress it up according to the best traditions of the ethics of care?

One possible objection might be that empathy seems to be missing the emotional involvement and commitment associated with compassion: in the way it is used in medicine empathy seems to be no more than a (superficial) technique. A closer look at the literature, however, shows that this objection is not too well informed. In the first place, there is much conceptual clarity about the concept of empathy, especially with respect to related concepts like sympathy and compassion (Stepien & Baernstein 2006). In the clinical context, empathy is more than understanding or appreciating how someone feels. It is considered to include emotive, moral, cognitive and behavioural dimensions. Some authors consider sympathy to be the same as the emotional component of empathy. Other authors see empathy as a multi-phase process rather than as a single event (Benbassat & Baumal 2004). According to Benbassat and Baumal empathy begins with gaining an insight into the patient's concerns, feelings and sources of distress. This is followed by engagement or identification with these feelings. Engagement produces compassion and compassion leads to a desire to alleviate the suffering or remove the case of distress.

The proposal to view empathy as a process has some interesting consequences. In the first place, it helps to get more grip on what takes place in the physician–patient relationship in terms of teachable components. Benbassat and Baumal believe that the ability to encourage the patient to convey his distress is a teachable skill. They give concrete advice about facilitating this first step. Secondly, we see compassion re-appearing at the heart of the process of empathy. Interestingly, however, in Benbassat's view compassion is produced by engagement, whereas according to Housset's analysis compassion just happens and might or might not result in engagement. Does this mean that we are talking about different meanings of compassion? Or is either one of the analyses mistaken?

The good thing about Benbassat's view is that he indentifies compassion as a core element in a clinical process of empathy, part of which can be promoted, measured and trained. Benbassat's practical view can be worked out further with suggestions made by Halpern who shows that empathy is not detached cognition, as it was taught in the 1960s, but emotional and nonverbal attunement that is rooted in ordinary communication (Halpern 2003). Housset's theoretical analysis refers to a different level: it helps in understanding the ethical meaning of compassion. Asking Benbassat and Halpern why compassion is important, they make clear that it is useful because it helps in appreciating the personal meanings of patients' words, in focusing and holding the physician's attention. It facilitates trust and disclosure and makes practicing medicine more meaningful. Asking Housset about the importance of compassion, his answer refers not to usefulness, but to the very structure of the way our ethical awareness is rooted in pre-moral emotions such as that of compassion.

Seeing that empathy is more than a technique, and understanding that according to many authors it does comprise compassion, what is our answer to the question whether or not "empathy can do the job?" We think it can be a qualified "yes". Looking for a more or less natural place for compassion in clinical medicine, empathy—if interpreted as a process comprising compassion—is a good starting point, because it connects with the already relatively strong position of the latter in medicine, without necessarily being reduced to a technique.

## 3. Conclusion: compassion and ethics of care

In this contribution we focused on the role of compassion in medical education. We agree with Housset that compassion is an important concept to be further developed in medical education. It helps in seeing the importance of a continuous critical hermeneutics of words, the possibility of compassion as a source of morality and the fact that compassion constitutes and reveals a form of community. We also placed some critical comments. Compassion can be silenced or sidelined by the impact of institutions. It can be threatened by excess and onesidedness. It can sometimes fall short, be completely absent, be sometimes falsely deemed to be there or it can be turned into disgust. Although further research on these subjects still waits to be done, we endorse the idea of using the concept of empathy as a good way of embedding compassion in medicine. How does all this relate to the ethics of care?

One way of establishing the relationship of compassion to the ethics of care is by relating the subject to the four stages of care as presented by Joan Tronto (1993). Determining the role of compassion in this process, it seems that compassion, in the sense of being "opened up" by someone else's need, is always there, right at the very beginning of the "caring about". The powerful thing about compassion is that it aligns with the original inspiration of many medical students. But we have also seen that if good care were dependent on compassion as a pre-moral spontaneous reaction, the very basis of care would depend too much on unpredictable emotional responses. Moreover, a great deal of medical ethical education should be about the development of the student's original inspiration. And we have also seen that in order to be sure that compassion has a solid position, one needs to be aware of, and offer resistance to, the systemic pressure inherent in health care institutions. Developing the original inspiration of compassion that is embedded in the already existing attention to empathy might meet these demands. In the best case, compassion can then, at once, play a role as a pre-moral emotion, as a moral emotion or virtue, and as a behavior, Housset helps us to see the value of compassion on a theoretical ethical level. Empathy might help us to root it in the reality of medical practice.

## Notes

[1] We do not mean that there is no interest in the formation of young physicians as communicative and sensitive doctors. In our country, and we assume the same is true for the rest of Europe, all medical schools provide training in communication skills. Some schools use films, literature and poetry to train and develop greater emotional sensitivity in medical practitioners. The point, however, is that this is not deliberately connected to the original inspiration and motivation of the students to choose this profession.

[2] Bertolami complains that there is a lot of teaching *about* ethics, which is not the same as teaching ethics.

[3] One of the professions Dubet discusses is the nursing profession that is made up of (and constantly threatened to be torn apart by) the logic of the reinforcement of scientific medicine, the logic of service and caring, and the logic of reinforcement of the patient's autonomy (195-230).

[4] Collier, reports that 23% of US medical residents thought they had become less humanistic during their training, and as many as 61% reported becoming more cynical.

[5] Although the content of the article has been cut to make it a shorter read because of the pressure of time on many physicians, in a personal communication Sulmasy confided that he has never had so much trouble trying to have an article published. Puchalsky claims that trained physicians only need two minutes to take a spiritual history according to her FICA-tool (Puchalsky 2002).

[6] Writing this section I learned much from a discussion with Rolf Ahlzen, physician and philosopher, Karlstad University, Sweden.

[7] For both a rich overview of recent literature and a critical discussion of the difficulties one meets promoting empathy: Shapiro 2008 (freely accessible at: http://www.peh-med.com/content/3/1/10, visited on 26 January 2009).

# 8.

# *The perspective of intellectual disability care on asymmetry in the care-relationship: towards empowering compassion*

Axel Liégeois

## 1. The assumptions of asymmetry and compassion

The assumptions of the research question are twofold: the asymmetry in the care-relationship and compassion to deal with this asymmetry. We elucidate these two assumptions.

### *Asymmetry in the care-relationship*

The first assumption is the fundamental tension between symmetry and asymmetry in the care-relationship (van Heijst 2005). On the one hand, this relationship is symmetric because both care-receivers and care-providers are equivalent persons. They are equivalent in respect of their human dignity. On the other hand, the relationship is asymmetric since there is definite imbalance of power in the relationship between unequal persons in an unequal position. The care-providers assume professional responsibility to provide high quality care. They have expert knowledge, adequate skills and good attitudes. The care-receivers, on the contrary, have a health or disability problem and cannot cope with it any more, even with the support of informal carers such as family members. Hence, the care-receivers are vulnerable and dependent on professional care-providers.

This creates an asymmetric relationship in which the person who provides care inevitably exercises power over the person who needs care. The asymmetry of power in the relationship is a structural and not a moral fact. It exists by virtue of the structure of the care relationship and precedes the moral action and interaction. Nevertheless, asymmetry is not only a relational, but also a social and political matter. The way care is actually organised in society predominantly enhances or improves the asymmetry in the relationship.

### *The concept of compassion*

Another assumption of this research is that the concept of compassion provides a way of dealing with the asymmetry in the care relationship. This concept has been developed in a creative way by Emmanuel Housset is his book *L'intelligence de la pitié. Phénoménologie de la communauté* (2003). We do not need to develop the concept of compassion extensively since Housset has written a chapter on the *Paradoxes of Pity* in the present book. In his book and in his chapter, he does not formulate a concise definition, but gives a broad description of what compassion is and is not.

Nevertheless, we need a working definition for our own research purposes. We propose to describe Housset's (2003) concept of compassion in a concise way "as the respectful awareness of being touched by the other person's suffering." We can work out this definition with the following elements: "Compassion arises in the mutual encounter of two persons. It presumes listening without judging and being empathic to the unique other. It is not a withdrawal in ones own feelings of compassion. It is a bodily, emotional and intelligent experience. It leads to a community of suffering. It appeals to take care of the suffering. And finally, compassion is a source of respect for the other." We add two other definitions of compassion. The *Oxford Dictionary* (2005) defines compassion as "a strong feeling of sympathy for people who are suffering and the desire to help them." In *Wikipedia. The Free Encyclopedia* (2007) compassion is described as "an understanding of the emotional state of another" and as "a desire to alleviate or reduce the suffering of another."

When we overview these definitions of compassion, we can discern two of its constitutive elements, namely the fact of being touched by the other person's suffering and the desire to alleviate this suffering.

## 2. The perspective of intellectual disability care

Can we use this concept of compassion to deal with the asymmetry in the care-relationship? We deal with this question from the specific perspective of professional care for people with intellectual disability. Especially in the care of these persons, the asymmetric relationship and the concept of compassion are delicate matters. The asymmetry seems greater since the intellectual disability causes important limitations on the person. This situation incites people to be more compassionate to a person with intellectual disability. The delicacy of this matter becomes yet clearer when we take into account the shift in attitude towards intellectual disability which started at the beginning of the 1990s. The shift was threefold: a shift in terminology, in definition and in paradigm.

### *Shift in terminology*

The traditional terminology consists of "mental retardation" and "mental handicap." Mental retardation is a more medical term that we find both in the *Diagnostic and Statistical Manual of Mental Disorders* (DSM-IV-TR, 2003), the internationally established manual of psychiatric diagnosis, and in the American Association of Mental Retardation, the leading organization in the field of mental disability. In this old terminology, mental disability is seen as a medical defect. And the disabled persons are totally identified with their defect: they are *the* "mentally retarded" or *the* "mentally handicapped."

Only since the beginning of 2007, has the AAMR officially become the AAIDD, the American Association on Intellectual and Developmental Disabilities. "Intellectual and developmental disability" and "people with intellectual and developmental disability" has become the new terminology. In this view, the persons are not identified with their disability, but are first of all human persons, who have secondly an intellectual and developmental disability with consequences for their functioning in the community.

We use the terms "intellectual disability" and "people with intellectual disability." Nevertheless, we are aware of the fact that the term "intellectual" refers to a disability that is not only intellectual and developmental, but embraces both the intellectual and the emotional development, for the intellectual limitation has important consequences for the emotional and affective life of the persons.

### *Shift in definition*

Parallel to the shift in terminology there has been a shift in definition. The old definitions of the AAMR, last repeated in the definition of 1983, stressed the intellectual functioning of the person, or the "significant sub-average of general intellectual functioning." This view is expressed in the old and probably well known classification of mental retardation or mental handicap in degrees of IQ, Intelligence Quotient. There is borderline mental retardation when the IQ is between 70 and 79. Mild mental retardation refers to an IQ of 50 to 69, and moderate mental retardation to an IQ of 35 to 49. In severe mental retardation the IQ is between 20 and 34 and in profound mental retardation the IQ refers to a level below 20.

Since 1992, the AAMR has adopted a new definition in which the stress is less on the intellectual functioning and more on the consequence: the position of the individual in the community. In the most recent definition of 2010, intellectual disability is defined as "a disability characterized by significant limitations, both in intellectual functioning and in adaptive behavior as expressed in conceptual, social, and practical skills; this disability originates before age 18" (AAIDD 2010; Schalock 2010; Vehmas 2004). In the official explanation of the definition, intellectual disability is not seen as something the person has, nor as something the person is. Intellectual disability is considered to be a state of functioning that reflects the "fit" between the capabilities of the person and the structure and expectations of the community.

### *Shift in paradigm*

A last shift concerns the paradigms, namely the shift from the defect-paradigm over the development-paradigm to the citizenship-paradigm (Greenspan 1999; van Gennep 2000). The defect-paradigm holds a medical view: the handicap is a defect, a disease or impairment. The development-paradigm has a special educational background: the handicap is a limitation in learning abilities that can be improved. The citizenship-paradigm is a based on a social critical point of view: the disability is the consequence of unequal rights and duties in the society.

In the defect-paradigm, the care consists of medical treatment, offered in the doctor-patient relationship, and has often been characterized by paternalism. In the development-paradigm, the relationship is that of a teacher and a pupil, and care aims mainly at education and training of the abilities. Finally in the citizenship-paradigm, all people are considered to be equal citizens with a right to quality of life, but some citizens need special support because of their intellectual disability.

In the first paradigm, the mentally retarded live in separate institutions, segregated from society. In the second paradigm, the handicapped are educated according to the principle of normalization, in special services in the community. In the third paradigm, people with disability should be able to use the normal services in the community.

### *The concept of empowerment*

In the citizenship-paradigm, the leading principle is empowerment of the people with intellectual disability. The *Oxford Dictionary* (2005) defines the verb empower as "to give somebody the power or authority to do something." In *Wikipedia* (2007) empowerment refers to "increasing the spiritual, political, social or economic strength of individuals and communities. It often involves the empowered developing confidence in their own capacities." For our own research purposes, we define empowerment as "the process of respecting the own choices of care-receivers in order to improve their control over the care and over their life."

The presumption of empowerment in the care for people with intellectual disability is the primacy of the community (van Gennep 2000). All people, with or without disability, are equal citizens. All of them should take part in community life. Hence disability is seen as the result of an excluding community. Citizens, therefore, should be ready to include people with intellectual disability into the community. For a real inclusion, equal opportunities are not enough, but equal outcomes are also required.

The aim of empowerment is to improve the quality of life of people with intellectual disability. Quality of life is the valuation of the functioning of the person in the community. It comprises several dimensions or domains of life, such as the physical, psycho-social and spiritual dimension. The valuation is mostly subjective by the person with intellectual disability. Nevertheless, some more objective, material conditions are necessary to improve quality of life. Of course, there are important cultural variations.

The means of empowerment is support. Because people with intellectual disability have limitations in their intellectual functioning and their adaptive behavior, they need special support to make choices and control their own life. Which support is given depends on the assessment of the special needs in the specific circumstances of the individual person with intellectual disability. It can be provided by people within the person's own social network or by professional care-providers.

### *A critical remark*

In our opinion, the citizenship-paradigm and its concept of empowerment are very idealistic. Although people with intellectual disability have significant limitations in their intellectual functioning and their adaptive behavior, they are seen as equal citizens with legal rights who participate in the community. The paradigm of citizenship and empowerment aligns with an individualistic view of the human person and a liberal concept of society. People with intellectual disability are seen as independent individuals who should have control over their own life. With some support, they should live nearly independently in the community and be productive in the free market economy.

The short-sightedness of this view seems very obvious when we look at the target group itself: this ideal is only suitable for people with a mild and moderate intellectual disability, and not for people with a severe or profound intellectual disability. They will never be able to participate in the community, to live in an independent way and to be productive in the society, even with the best support, because they are too limited in their intellectual functioning and adaptive behaviour. In our opinion, the stress in the definition of intellectual disability moves too much from the limitations of the person to the inclusion in the community. The limitations caused by intellectual disability are nevertheless undeniable.

## 3. A critical reflection on compassion

Now we develop a critical view on the concept of compassion from the perspective of intellectual disability care. We first make a critical reflection on this concept, influenced by our praxis as ethicist in the care for people with intellectual disability. Then we check our reflection against that of professional care-providers by means of a short inquiry that we set up.

### *A critical reflection on compassion*

We have described the important turn from a defect-paradigm over the development-paradigm towards the citizenship-paradigm. It is clear that from the perspective of the new paradigm, the word "compassion" is to be identified with the old paradigms. Above we defined compassion as the fact of being touched by the other person's suffering and the desire to alleviate this suffering. In compassion the subjects are the care-providers who are touched and who desire to give care, while the care-receivers are suffering people and objects of this care.

From the perspective of the citizenship-paradigm, compassion tends to paternalism. The care-providers have compassion and help the care-receivers for their benefit. The care-providers make decisions on the care-receivers' behalf, without respecting the care-receivers' choices enough and without giving them control over their own life. From the perspective of the citizenship-paradigm, compassion is identified with an exaggerated tendency to help people with intellectual disability effectively rendering them helpless. It seems to be the contrary of empowerment. This criticism of the old defect- and development-paradigms is not only scientifically founded in social criticism, but is also a very emotional reaction against human experience of segregation, humiliation and abuse. Consequently, we think that the word compassion will not be given a high evaluation by today's professional care-providers.

### *The design of the inquiry*

To put our personal reflection on trial, we carried out a short inquiry among professional care-providers. This inquiry does not claim scientific validity, but is a limited critical touchstone of our personal opinion. In the inquiry, we asked twelve professional care-providers, working in the field of care for people with intellectual disability and participating in the Ethics Committee of the Brothers of Charity, to answer a questionnaire consisting of three questions.

The first question concerned appreciation of the word "compassion." Because the participants speak Dutch, the word "medelijden" was presented, with the explicit mention that it is the translation of the English word "compassion." The participants could score on a scale from 1 to 10 and could give further comments.

In the next question appreciation of the concept of empowerment was verified. The word empowerment was presented to the participants, together with the Dutch translation of the definition we mentioned above: "Empowerment is the process of respecting the own choices of people with intellectual disability and of giving them control over their own life." The participants could score on a scale from 1 to 10 and could give further comments.

The final question related to the appreciation of the concept of compassion. Here the word compassion was neither mentioned nor suggested. We presented to the participants the Dutch translation of our above mentioned concise description of Housset's concept of compassion: "A respectful awareness of being touched by the other person's suffering. It arises in the mutual encounter of two persons. It presumes listening without judging and being empathic to the unique other. It is not a withdrawal in one's own feelings of compassion.

It is a bodily, emotional and intelligent experience. It leads to a community of suffering. It appeals to take care of the suffering. And finally, it is a source of respect for the other." Again, the participants could score on a scale from 1 to 10 and could give further comments.

All participants filled in the questionnaire completely and anonymously. The inquiry does not claim scientific validity, but is a welcome trial of our personal opinion.

### *Results and discussion*

Our critical reflection is largely confirmed by the results of the inquiry. The first question concerned the appreciation of the word "compassion." This receives a score of 42 out of 100. That is not so bad, taking into account the critical reflection we developed above from the perspective of intellectual disability care. In their comments, the participants appreciate that suffering is seen as a part of life and that one can be touched by another's suffering. But the participants deprecate compassion as too emotional an experience. For some participants, compassion is considered to be a humiliation of people with intellectual disability and not to show enough respect for them. In their opinion, compassion is a subjective feeling that needs the active complement of professional care. These critical comments partially correspond to the ideas of Housset who rejects "fake compassion", "malivola benevolentia" and compassion as "egoism in disguise" (2003). This proves that it is absolutely necessary to develop a profound criticism of the word compassion.

It is remarkable that the concept of compassion, as described in the inquiry, receives a higher evaluation. Without using the word compassion and without knowing that the description refers to Housset's concept of compassion, the participants give this concept a score of 85 out of 100. In the concept of compassion, the participants appreciate the mutual encounter, the listening and empathising without judging, the respect for the dignity of the person and the appeal to the other. But they also find that compassion has a too pessimistic view on human life, because it emphasises suffering. They prefer a more optimistic view that includes also sharing the joy of life. And once again, compassion needs the active complement of professional care.

Finally, the word empowerment and its description receive an evaluation of 80 out of 100. From the perspective of our critical reflection, it is remarkable that the appreciation of empowerment is not higher than that of compassion. It is even a little lower, namely 80 for empowerment and 85 for compassion.

A remarkable conclusion of the inquiry is that the concept of compassion scores twice as much as the word compassion, namely 85 versus 42 out of 100. Therefore, it seems very useful to look for a new word that takes into account the criticisms of the concept, but especially of the word "compassion."

### *Alternative words for compassion?*

There are several synonyms for compassion. One of them is empathy, a well-known word in care. It was introduced by Carl Rogers in Client-Centred Therapy. He defines empathy as the ability "to perceive the internal frame of reference of another with accuracy and with the emotional components and meanings which pertain thereto as if one were the person, but without ever losing the 'as if' condition" (Rogers 1959, 210-211). Empathy expresses an important element of compassion, namely the strong feeling of sympathy for the suffering person, but without the desire to help the other person. Moreover, empathy has become a technical term in the domain of counseling and psychotherapy. Therefore, it is not the best word to express the more ethical idea of compassion.

Another synonym for compassion is sympathy. This term is free of psychotherapeutic connotations. It has exactly the same meaning and etymology as compassion, namely to share the suffering with the other. Dorothee Sölle defined sympathy as "the ability to be touched by the other person's suffering and the growing power to fight against injustice" (1979, back flap). In our opinion, it is a very good definition because both constitutive elements of compassion are mentioned, namely the being touched by the other person's suffering and the desire to alleviate this suffering. Sympathy in its original meaning and as understood by Sölle seems to be the best synonym of compassion. Unfortunately, the actual word sympathy does not express any more the rich meaning of the original Greek word or Sölle's concept. Maybe today the word sounds too "sympathetic."

## 4. An integrative approach

Because the search for an alternative word for compassion does not seem to be very fruitful, we look for another approach. We try to integrate both the perspective of disability and the concept of empowerment on the one hand, and the concept of compassion on the other hand. The key to this integrative approach is the link between compassion and asymmetry in care.

### *The perspective of intellectual disability care*

In the assumptions of this research, we described the symmetry and asymmetry in the care-relationship. The care-relationship is symmetric because both care-providers and care-receivers are equivalent persons in respect to their human dignity. At the same time, the relationship is asymmetric since there is an imbalance of power in the relationship between two unequal persons, namely care-providers who are competent in professional care and care-receivers who are vulnerable and dependent of professional care. We qualified this power relationship as structural and not as a moral fact.

In the critical reflection on compassion from the perspective of intellectual disability care, we suggested that the word compassion is identified with the paradigms of defect and development. Moreover, compassion tends to paternalism. This means that care-providers would make decisions on the care-receivers' behalf, but without giving enough respect to their choices. From the point of view of the citizenship-paradigm, the care-providers would fail in their duty to empower the care-receivers. Care-providers should support care-receivers in making choices in order to improve their control over their own life.

When we now make the link between compassion and asymmetry from the point of view of the citizenship-paradigm, we can state that compassion tends to foster the asymmetry in the care relationship. Asymmetry in the care relationship is inevitably a structural fact. It precedes the moral act. The asymmetry becomes a moral matter when the care-providers take advantage of or exploit this asymmetry. Ethics concerns the way people deliberately deal with the asymmetry. According to the citizenship-paradigm, compassion is a deliberate confirmation of the structural asymmetry in the care relationship. Care-providers should, on the contrary, compensate the asymmetry. This is precisely what the citizenship-paradigm means by empowerment. Care-providers should compensate the power in the structural care relationship by empowering the care-receiver. They should strive for a better balance of power or to equalize power by giving the other *more* power. Empowerment is thus an ethical duty of care-providers. Compassion seems to be the opposite, namely a confirmation of the power in the structural care-relationship.

### *The perspective of care ethics*

From the perspective of care ethics, we find that compassion is misunderstood by the citizenship-paradigm. Nevertheless, we should be open to these critical remarks. They offer a constructive contribution to a better understanding of compassion. In our opinion, care ethics should integrate this critical view.

From our personalist view, we see care ethics as a relational approach in which the human person is basically related to others (Liégeois 2008; 2009). In our opinion, the defect- and development-paradigms and the citizenship-paradigm are one-sided and individualistic. They consider either the care-providers or the care-receiver to be independent individuals who make their own choices and appeal to their own responsibility. The defect- and development-paradigms stress the responsibility of the care-providers at the risk of their making choices in a paternalistic way. The citizenship-paradigm, on the contrary, emphasizes the care-receivers' own responsibility at the risk of reducing the care-providers to the implementation of the care-receivers' choices. In a personalist view on care ethics the relational dimension of human existence should be applied consequentially to a mutual partnership in care. It is neither up to the care-providers nor to the care-receivers to make choices and to appeal to their own responsibility. Both of them are involved in a mutual partnership with a process of joint choice-making and shared responsibility.

In this personalist view on care ethics, it should be possible to relate the positive elements of compassion to the positive criticism of empowerment. Integration should be possible. Because we did not find an alternative word for compassion, we propose to create a new concept in which we combine compassion and empowerment. This combination is supported by the inquiry in which both concepts have a high appreciation, namely 85 to 100 for compassion and 80 to 100 for empowerment.

### *Towards empowering compassion*

We therefore propose the new concept of "empowering compassion." In this word combination, "compassion" is the noun; "empowering" is the adjective. "Compassion" refers to the disposition and "empowering" to the action. This aligns with the classic ethical analysis of human action, which consists of an inner act, disposition or virtue, and an outer act or behavior (Janssens 1972). The disposition is the motivation, the driving motor or inspiring source of the action.

In this new concept, Housset's description is still the reference for the positive elements of compassion. Compassion is the respectful awareness of being touched by the other person's suffering. It arises in the mutual encounter of two persons. It presumes listening without judging and being empathic to the unique other. It is not a withdrawal into one's own feelings of compassion. It is a bodily, emotional and intelligent experience. It leads to a community of suffering.

Where compassion could be misunderstood from the perspective of the citizenship-paradigm, we add the positive element of empowerment. We also adjust the too liberal element of empowerment by emphasizing the element of mutual relationship in care ethics. Empowering compassion thus makes the appeal to take care of the other's suffering. The disposition motivates to action. Compassion invites care that empowers. In this care, empowering compassion develops a mutual partnership between care-provider and care-receiver. In this partnership, the care-provider respects as much as possible the care-receiver's own choices in order to improve his or her control over the care and over his or her life.

## 5. Conclusion

We started this article with the research question whether we can use the concept of compassion to deal with the asymmetry in the care relationship. We gave a response from the specific perspective of professional care for people with intellectual disability in which empowerment is a key-concept. Our conclusion is that the new concept of empowering compassion is in fact able to deal in an ethical way with the inevitable structural asymmetry of the care relationship. On the one hand, empowering compassion is aware of the asymmetry because of the unequal position of care-provider and care-receiver. On the other hand, empowering compassion strives for symmetry and equal power because both persons deserve equal dignity. Empowering compassion starts from an unequal position in which one person suffers and the other doesn't, but both of them grow into a community of suffering and care, where empowerment alleviates the suffering. Empowering compassion is thus the respectful awareness of being touched by the other's suffering and the growing empowerment to alleviate this suffering.

# 9.

# Justice, care and (the) recognition (of dependency and vulnerability)

Christa Schnabl

The need to receive care and the necessity of giving care, two very important aspects of modern societies, have become a topic of discussion in recent years and are under construction today. In traditional settings women were one of the most important providers of care but in the last twenty years the situation has changed in various ways. The growth of women's participation in education and in the labour market has led to a new situation. Time constraints and their responsibilities in the labour market are limiting the hours women have available to care for children and the elderly. Women are no longer the only, nor the main group of people responsible for giving care and for meeting the need for care in modern societies. Migrants, for example, have become important care workers nowadays.

Consequently new questions have been raised in order to manage these recent developments—questions which deal with the problem of justice regarding the system of care in modern societies. How can care and care work be organized in a just and suitable manner? How can people who deal with care be treated in a just way? How should care and care work be valued and be recognized in modern societies which tend to use care work as an indispensable but free resource? Who should practice care and which conditions should be established to practice care and to organize care in our societies?

This article deals with questions of care and justice in modern ethical theories and focuses particularly on the value of recognition in this context. Can recognition and recognition theories help to improve the value of care and to establish care relations in a just manner?

Estelle Ferrarese argues that she is optimistic that recognition (recognition theories) helps us to focus on human vulnerability better and to derive rights from this principle of vulnerability. From my point of view, in fact, I am not so optimistic, and I am not convinced that recognition helps us integrate vulnerability better. May be that recognition can help theoretically, but if you consider Axel Honneth's theory of recognition, I have some practical doubts which derive from the detail of his view on care.

Moreover, I'm not a specialist in recognition theories but I did do some research in care-ethics. I wrote a book about "caring in a fair, just, and righteous way" (Schnabl 2005). My special focus is—as in my field of expertise—care and social ethics. The question I therefore raise is how we can give care and care relations their rightful place within the context of ethics and politics, a place which care and care relations need to have for the benefit of individual and social life in late modern society. In this context, at the very beginning, I want to stress that justice is an important category within this question too and we have to make sure that care solutions are good, righteous and just for both care-givers and care-receivers despite their different concerns. Therefore, we have to acknowledge justice as an inevitable and normative idea for our social order. My special view is the perspective of care-ethics. Therefore my focus will be the evaluation of the moral significance of the concepts of "recognition" in relation to a/symmetry within care situations and to reconsider "recognition" from an "ethics of care" point of view.

The topic of particular interest to me is whether the concept of recognition, especially Honneth's concept of recognition, has moral significance; on the one hand, for care-situations in particular and, on the other hand, for care-situations in our societies. Hence, I want to revise the significance of recognition in order to look at the consequences of recognition by pointing out Honneth's conception of care.

I will start by saying that, first of all, I'm very keen on Honneth´s conception of recognition. His sensibility towards new ethical questions and challenges beyond the Kantian Moral Philosophy paradigm is praiseworthy. Honneth is one of the male contemporary moral philosophers (e.g. in the German context), who has taken notice of the care-debate in feminist ethics since the 1980s and who pursues the integration of aspects of care-ethics in his moral theory (Bohmeyer 2008). Despite this, a second view in his texts (especially his texts about care) makes clear that there are difficulties with integrating asymmetry and asymmetric forms of care in this concept, especially within the horizon of justice, because Honneth develops a great gap between care/care-relations and justice. His theoretical framework of the three levels of recognition does not allow him to integrate care and justice. If care cannot be combined with justice on a fundamental level, there is no possibility of integrating care in a socio-ethical view of modern society. To sum up my argument at the beginning: I´m in favour of recognition in a Honnethian sense. My understanding of recognition in his sense is that it is *one* single element that is necessary to legitimate moral philosophy in general (in order to get a real-life or phenomenological foundation of morality). However, there is no special foundation-quality in Honneth's concept of recognition which would legitimate care, care relations or asymmetry in a specific way. The link between recognition, care and justice should be drawn in a more explicit way, more explicit than Honneth tried to. More than recognition in a broader sense, I want to stress the recognition of vulnerability as a special kind of dependency and need, a recognition which is necessary in order to understand care, care-ethics and care relations better. Let me point out, step by step, three aspects that underline my argument.

First, I want to introduce Honneth's theory and his topic of recognition. Second, I'll describe the consequences of Honneth's theory on care and care-relations. Third, I want to describe my own position on this subject matter.

## 1. Honneth's "theory of recognition"

First we have to consider the content of Honneth's recognition theory and his thinking on care (Honneth 2000, 133). Honneth wants to point out the borders of modern moral philosophy while he stresses that postmodern ethics gives an innovative, new input. Modern philosophy theories are too focused on a universalistic approach without sensibilities towards individual and special situations. Modern ethics approaches (in which justice is the central value) are not, by definition, able to integrate this perspective of uniqueness. Therefore we need alternatives, which do not broaden the aspect of justice, but reflect the point of distinctive otherness or human care. Symmetry and the moral point of view, which deal with equal treatment (Ger: *Gleichbehandlung*) have to be adjusted and corrected. We have to integrate the moral duty of responsibility for others, who need help in different kinds of situations. This specific form of relationship among humans cannot be subsumed in our equality theories, because these care relationships are asymmetric. Such kinds of obligation cannot be included in categories of equal treatment. Due to postmodern ethics this new form of duty results in a challenge for further development in ethics. Keeping this idea in mind, we have to transcend the normative horizon of modernity, not only enlarge it.

This now brings me to my next point. In order to deal with this postmodern ethical challenge, Honneth, in his text *The Other of Justice*, proposes to reconceptualize the obligation of care. He describes it in terms of Levinas' Antlitz (Fr: *Visage*):

> If this optical process is described genuinely enough, then it should become evident that the experience of an ethical demand is also always given in such an event. At the sight of the „face" (Ger: *Antlitz*, Fr: *visage*) of another person, we have no choice but to help this person immediately and to assist him or her in coping with existential problems. (Honneth 2007a, 119; 2000, 161)

In Levinas' perspective, ethical obligation is grounded in the perception of the Visage of the Other. Honneth himself combines this concept with his own philosophical system of recognition. This transformation process results in essential variances e.g. in the concept of symmetry and asymmetry. On a phenomenological level Honneth stresses the high significance of recognition for the baby and the child. But not only do children need recognition to develop a healthy identity and a stable character, all human beings need recognition in different ways. Honneth, when quoting Dewey, makes a significant point:

> every rational understanding of the world is always already bound up with a holistic form of experience, in which all elements of a given situation are qualitatively disclosed from a perspective of engaged involvement. If we follow this train of thought far enough, it becomes possible not only to make a transition from the notion of "care" to that of "recognition" but also to demonstrate the primacy of this kind of recognition over all merely cognitive attitudes toward the world. (Honneth 2005a, 110; 2005b, 40)

Beyond this phenomenological level, recognition also includes the aspect of normative significance. In this respect recognition means a specific form of consciousness about the world and self-consciousness of oneself. As an affirmative attitude which others provide for the self, it would be primary to all other forms of world relationship (Ger: *Weltverhältnis*) such as, for example, cognition. Recognition implies an affirmative, existentialistic attitude of caring. All other forms of perception of the world are consequences and derive from this primary form of qualitative union between oneself and the other. Furthermore, Honneth stresses the reciprocal form of mutual recognition. This leads him to his position in 'Kampf um Anerkennung', which describes the mother and the baby as mutually reciprocally dependent on each other in the very first couple of months of the new life (Honneth 1992, 161). One could think that Honneth's bizarre position might lead to an imbalance of mother-child dependency.

On a basic level I partly agree with Honneth's consideration of the significance of recognition for the foundation of morality. Recognition is the basis for one's capacity to act and it is the philosophical grounding for his theory of recognition and the three levels: love, law and solidarity. Secondly, I agree with Honneth's concern that economic discrimination/disadvantage, as well as cultural deprivation, are different types of social injustice and both are rooted in a kind of denied/refused recognition. According to Honneth and in opposition to Nancy Fraser, I want to say that on a basic, and on the very theoretical, level we need not operate with two different normative values, namely redistribution and recognition (Fraser & Honneth 2003). It is quite possible to derive both from one theoretical root. But for an application in concrete political fields, I agree with Fraser (contrary to Honneth) on the pluralism in practical principles needed to change our social circumstances effectively.

## 2. Consequences of the recognition-approach for care relations and care-ethics

After saying that recognition is important for our justification of ethics, I now want to turn to the second part of my article, in which I discuss the question of whether recognition has an influence on caring, on the ethics of care or on conceptualizing asymmetric relations of caring in a specific way. I´m raising this question because we have to consider the specific significance of recognition for caring, for care-ethics and care-politics (e.g. to increase the importance of care relationships in our society).

First, I want to follow Honneth's position and will describe how Honneth integrates care into his ethical concept, before I provide my own position on this subject matter. What consequences does Honneth´s ethical justification of recognition have for his re-placement of care? Can we see an adequate fit of care-relations in ethics and politics? Are there any visible consequences for the problem of asymmetric ethical duty in dependency relationships when caring for the other?

I would like to start by arguing on the level of principle once more: Honneth stresses (as I pointed out at the beginning) the significance of care for the further development of ethics.

> What has been said so far, however, must also be accompanied by the conclusion that care be again awarded that place in the domain of the moral which it has all to frequently been denied in the Kantian tradition of moral philosophy. Just as solidarity constitutes a necessary counterpoint to the principle of justice inasmuch as it furnishes the affective impulses of reciprocal recognition in a particularistic manner, care represents its equally necessary counterpoint, because it supplements this

> principle of justice with a principle of unilateral, entirely disinterested help (Honneth 2007a, 125; 2000, 170).

What this now means is that care is a necessary complement to justice, because it supplements justice with the principle of one sided, completely uninterested help. Now, what is the right ethical position for caring? Honneth proposes caring to be quite in opposition to autonomy and justice. He describes his position using Levinas` figure of the visage, but in a different way from Levinas. (It is, more or less, a re-reading of Levinas). While Levinas´ caring-obligation constitutes the core of justice, meaning that concern for others is the crucial sense or the principal item of justice, Honneth points out:

> Because of the sight of the face of another person I am said to have no choice but to feel obligated to care for this person, I must be aware that I am restricted in my individual autonomy and that my own interests are only of subordinate significance (Honneth 2007a, 119; 2000, 162).

As you can see in this sentence, caring is a complete one-way action, a consequence of a non-reciprocal devotion. This action can limit one´s own autonomy (meaning the autonomy of the care-giver) to a great extent. This perspective of care results in a tension between care and justice as well as in a form of ethical dualism, which can be described with the following comparison:

| Justice | Care |
|---|---|
| Observation of law | Unlimited, unending benevolence |
| Obligation to equal treatment | Asymmetric obligation, to act in favour of benevolence towards the individual other |
| Equal rights in a formal sense | Perception of the uniqueness |
| Autonomy | Heteronomy |
| Symmetrical relationship | Asymmetrical relationship |

For Honneth, there is no possibility of transcending from one side of action or ethical logic to the other. The ethical principles of the two systems are incompatible and incongruous. There is no other superior ethical idea, which can open a perspective which combines care and justice. Care and justice mark a conflict, which cannot be solved. From its genesis, the principle of care is a primary one, because it stands at the beginning of the development of each child. All other developments including the development of morality follow this kind of relationship. Furthermore, it is not only a relationship of genetical primacy, but also a relationship of mutual normative incompatibility.

This consequence provides a care-justice antagonism for our normative conception of morality. While care embodies the logic of self-abandonment, justice focuses on the logic of balancing equal claims of self-interested individuals. Care is an asymmetric obligation, tending towards the unlimited uniqueness of the individual other. It is a completely one-sided and non-reciprocal phenomenon. This form of obligation, which results from the care perspective, might restrain autonomy to a great extent. Furthermore, this picture of care and care obligation leads to a restricted form of care-reasonability (I mean "Zumutbarkeit" in the German language). The imperative to care for others calls for action from the care-giver, who should care for the person next to him—or her—self. One might not be surprised that this person is often a female person.

To put this in Honneth's words: Between justice and care persists

> not only a relation of genetic primacy but also one of reciprocal exclusiveness: an obligation to care and to be benevolent can only exist when a person is in such an extreme state of need and hardship that the moral principle of equal treatment can no longer be applied in a balanced manner. Therefore, human beings who are either physically or mentally unable to participate in practical discourses deserve at least the selfless care of those who are emotionally bound to them. But, conversely, the moment the other person is recognized as an equal being among all others – in that he or she is capable of participating in practical discourses – the unilateral relation of care must come to an end, for an attitude of benevolence is not permissible towards subjects who are able to articulate their beliefs and views publicly (Honneth 2007a, 124; 2000, 169).

I would like to stress that Honneth's notion on the attitude to welfare is a very powerful, striking argument which cannot be ignored and which calls for constructive criticism. Honneth's notion of care is based on a mutual exclusion between help and autonomy, between the need for help and independence. This mutual exclusion is directed at the care-giver as well as at the care-receiver. As soon as someone takes care of somebody else, one cannot speak of autonomy any longer. To receive care from someone means that one is dependent on the other person in a fundamental sense: for example one is unable to speak or unable to act autonomously. On the other hand: human beings have to demonstrate their fundamental inability, if they want others to recognize their need for care. In order to define the boundary between care and autonomy, Honneth stresses the ability to speak and the possibility of participating in discourse. Therefore the justified need for care presupposes an inability to speak. One can apply this criterion of necessity of care only in the case of some kind of severe illness or inability, but not in an everyday care situation. The boundaries between the ability to live autonomously and the need for help are often not so clear and explicit; imagine for example the care situation with children or with elderly people in the case of dementia. A strict boundary is problematic, especially from the political ethics perspective, because it means, that people who need help may not participate in political affairs. The consequence of this position in a strict sense is that people who need care cannot participate in public discourse.

Apart from the practical problem of defining the boundaries, another problem arises, namely the problem of defining the potential caregiver. We have to raise the question: who is obliged to care? Honneth confines the duty as an obligation for human beings who live with people in need and have strong emotions and deep personal relationships with them. I think, in this context you can surely imagine the strong connection between care and emotion as well as care and affective bonds. In this regard care is not a duty in general, but rather an obligation for people who share emotional bonds with the care-receivers. Therefore one has to ask the question, if care is compulsory only for close people. If we follow Honneth's position, we cannot make it legitimate that institutions, on the one hand, or men, on the other hand, should enter a care-obligation too. In this regard, we have had to clarify the question of care in a fair, just, and righteous way in a broader social context. However, Honneth's concept avoids this perspective, because he places care only on the level of love. A feminist approach has to visualize this implicit androcentric perspective, because it is usually women who establish the bonding and who know how to help. It cannot be fair that people who have fewer emotional bonds are less obliged to take care of others. In the end socialization only would be the most important criteria for caregiving. In this regard, care tends to be reduced to a kind of principle for only severe cases of need and inability when the ethics of equal treatment fail.

## 3. Is Honneth's concept of recognition morally relevant to the ethics of care? Some important elements for a socio-ethical theory of care.

I think that recognition in this regard doesn't make very much sense. The concept of recognition in the Honnethian sense is both too broad and too narrow at the same time.

On the one hand, it is too broad because recognition constitutes morality in general, but it doesn't constitute care in particular. This means that the focus of care ethics is not on how to preserve one's personal integrity but on how to care for people in need, under right and just circumstances, which neither lead to discrimination for caregivers nor for care-receivers.

On the other hand this concept is at the same time too narrow, because the privatization, the feminization and the emotionalization of care can neither be solved nor overcome. The asymmetrical form of recognition and the obligation to care is restricted by Honneth's love-level. The asymmetrical duty seems to be a duty only for family members.

Let me make a further restriction here. Recognition can help us to understand the individual care situation better. It makes people aware of, understanding of, and sensitive to the fact that we are all dependent on recognition. Recognition seems to be a category for the individual dimension of moral theory. However I do not notice any progression of care ethics in the sense of re-positioning care and care relationships in our society, if we integrate recognition and care in his/this regard.

Let me underline this argument and my proposal to make a correction to this concept: I think that in the concept of recognition, the mutual and symmetric form of recognition is ultimately dominated (explicit at level two and three). Therefore the asymmetric aspect of recognition is lost. From the perspective of care it is not only necessary but our duty to reintegrate this asymmetric dimension. To make a little correction in this matter: we have to realize the special forms of dependency in people who need care and in people who give care in families or institutions. Thereby, vulnerability (not in the sense of general but particular vulnerability) and one-way dependency, as a special kind of relationship, could serve as the missing link and the bridging element between care and recognition. This way of bridging draws attention to the asymmetric aspect of care and care situations. It is important to stress the fact that we are all potentially vulnerable, but in fact there are some who are crucially vulnerable. Not only are care-receivers vulnerable and dependent, but also care-givers who have to be sensitive to people in need. Care-givers don't look out for their own benefit but for the needs of the care-receivers. Therefore care-givers are vulnerable and dependent on a secondary derivative level. Eva Feder Kittay calls this level the second dependency of care-givers. What we now need is a reflection not only on vulnerability (as an existential dimension of human life) but also on dependency as a social reality and a special kind of relationship among people. To accept vulnerability (on the existential level) and dependency (on the social level) as unavoidable attributes of human life, in a special form but not only at the beginning and the end of life, is the challenge from the care-ethics perspective in particular.

My question is how we can raise care, vulnerability and asymmetrical duties onto a social and political level (Schnabl 2004; 2005;

2008). Vulnerability and recognition of vulnerability are conditions according to our anthropology of vulnerable human beings; they generate attitudes and virtues of recognition corresponding to the physical fact of vulnerability. In political ethics we often argue that solidarity is the modern value which describes the former duties of care in traditional societies. In my perspective, solidarity focuses on components other than care. Solidarity can be conceptualized as a symmetric or asymmetric obligation. In contrast, care in its classical version is always and only an asymmetric action which focuses on the benevolence of others. While solidarity reacts to forms of injustice caused by human beings, care responds to the needs of others, reflecting the existential fact that all human beings are born and have to die. Therefore we have to integrate this fact in our social theories to overcome the dualism of care and justice.

To bring care into the case of social ethics we have to reconceptualize care on three levels. On the first level, care can be defined as an obligation among family members, among people in love and in the family context, a form of reasonability which corresponds to the condition of emotional bonds. On this level, justice is relevant too because the practical realization of care has to be just and reasonable for care-givers and care-receivers. On the second level, care can be defined as a social virtue in the context of neighborhood and civil society but not in a strong sense of a moral obligation. On the third level, care has to be defined as a fundamental "human right" for people who need support for daily activities, in families as well as in institutions, in the case of unemployment, need, illness and disability. In correlation to the right to receive care we also have to focus on the right to give care without care-givers experiencing exclusion or discrimination.

# 10.

# *The shared premises of the ethics of care and theories of recognition: Vulnerability as moral category*

Estelle Ferrarese

"Micrological approach" was the term Theodor W. Adorno used to describe the attention to singularity, detail and the everyday which informed the thought of Walter Benjamin as it did his own (Adorno 1983, 236). Deriving from a philosophical posture constituted in the refusal of the primacy of the universal, it supposes that the particular is read at all times in the light of the painful contradiction between itself and the universal, between the system and the fragment. Furthermore, it signifies attentiveness to suffering and its subtle expressions, to the cries of pain which remain imperceptible to idealist systems. Hence the importance attributed by Adorno—as by Horkheimer—to this "other" of justice which is pity, a theme that runs through all of their writings. The *Dialectic of Enlightenment* admits that by reserving the responsibility of canceling injustice to fortuitous love of one's neighbor, pity accepts as unalterable the law of universal alienation which it would like to mitigate, however the same work also insists heavily on the fact that abandoning pity is tantamount to unburdening the individual of his moral intuitions.

Traces of this micrological approach which characterizes the first generation of the Frankfurt School are still visible in the theory of recognition as expounded by its current representatives, in particular Axel Honneth. It is these traces which legitimize a questioning of the possible convergence of the logic of recognition and that of care.

That said, my intention here is not to reduce care to pity, or even to compassion or benevolence. It is very clear that, for its defenders, this same term subsumes many meanings all at once: attitude and work (Kittay 1999, 30), affect and activity (Tronto 1987, 648). Regarding this second, material, physical, painful and sociological dimension of care, the Hegelian theories of recognition which I shall be concerned with here have quite simply nothing to say. From this point of view, in reality, the theories of care force a questioning of the material reality of recognition; Honneth has for example made numerous allusions to the need to reintroduce the world of things as well as the body into the theory of interaction; yet he draws no real conclusion as to the possible physical, tangible or technical dimension of recognition. Elucidating this undeniable blind spot of theories of recognition is however beyond the scope of this article; here, I shall be focusing on the common ground shared by the two bodies of theory, hence narrowing the problematic of care to its dimension of attitude.

Between these bodies of theory there of course exist crossovers and reciprocal commentary, however, as I shall demonstrate, in itself this is not sufficient to establish a real convergence. Rather, I believe that it is in an anthropology of vulnerability and the ethical preoccupations which stem from it that one can discern a commonality of viewpoints.

## 1. What the theory of recognition says about care

It must first of all be pointed out that the theorists of recognition have shown a marked and early interest for the theme of care and the debates which its sudden appearance in the philosophical field have given rise to. This is true of Axel Honneth in the first instance.

On the one hand, in a paper entitled "The Other of Justice: Habermas and the ethical challenge of postmodernism," Honneth discussed different attempts to bring a concern with the concrete particularity of persons and groups to the center of moral theory, among which Derrida's efforts to develop an ethics of asymmetrical obligation, and Carol Gilligan's theory of care. He acknowledges that this kind of ethics is the only non-assimilable challenge to moral theories of the Kantian sort: "The moral point of view of equal treatment [...]

requires continuous correction and supplementation by a viewpoint indebted to our concrete obligation to individual subjects in *need of help*." (Honneth 1995b, 291)

On the other hand, since *The Struggle for Recognition*, Honneth has carried out a tripartition of the possible forms of recognition, which correspond schematically to the self confidence which affective recognition brings within relationships of love, or even of friendship; the self respect which the legal recognition of one's belonging to a community of free beings brings; and the sense of self esteem which the social recognition of one's particular value brings.

The first is structured by the experience of the "affectionate attention of concrete others" (Honneth 1995a, 87). Recognition in this affective sphere implies taking the Other into consideration as unique, non-substitutable *and* a being of need: "Undisputed is a first, at least genetically, level on which subjects relate to themselves in such a way that they conceive of their physical needs and desires as a part of their own person that can be articulated." (Honneth 2005, 49) As a result, there exist duties of emotional assistance which extend, symmetrically or asymmetrically, to all partners of a primary relationship of this type; the typical case of an asymmetrical obligation being the relation parents have with their children; the typical case of a reciprocal obligation being the relation of friendship. Here Honneth identifies a normativity specific to love which appears to fit less into the Kantian moral tradition than into that of the ethics of care.

Admittedly, the recognition which occurs in the first sphere is not limited to a proven and enacted care. Following the work of psychoanalytic theorists such as Winnicott, Honneth believes that the formation of the subject takes place in this sphere when both mother and infant struggle against their initial symbiosis in order to achieve independence from each other. (Honneth 1995a, 96, 98, 105).

Yet, the (in-the-making) subject who appears here is presented in his incompleteness and his neediness; to the extent where Honneth conceives of moral progress in the sphere of love (his theory of recognition is firmly founded on a philosophy of history) in the form of "a step-by-step elimination of the role-clichés, stereotypes and cultural ascriptions that structurally impede adaptation to *others' needs*." (Honneth/Fraser 2003, 188. My emphasis) On that basis, the form which the gesture and the attitude of recognition must take in this sphere has a lot to do with what the theories of care have branded "*attentiveness*," which refers to an ability to perceive and respond to a need or a suffering. Joan Tronto equates its absence with "ignorance," describing it as "as a form of moral evil." (Tronto 1993, 127)

Similarly, it is worth noting that Jürgen Habermas does not imperiously evacuate "the Other" of the justice which his theory of communication focuses on. His curiosity for this "Other," a fossil leftover in his theory by a tradition which he progressively distanced himself from on many themes, first manifested itself in the form of an attention to pity.

He mentions pity at regular intervals, and not as an aberration, while admitting the absence of the mutual exclusion of pity and justice: "The reconciling power of compassion does not stand in opposition to the galvanizing power of rebellion against a world devoid of atonement and reparation for injustice. Solidarity and justice are two sides of the same coin," he concedes for example in an article on Horkheimer. (Habermas 1991, 134)

Given these resurgences, his model of impartial moral judgment, assuming the abstraction of the involved parties' motives, concrete circumstances, and existing institutions and life forms, finds itself placed in competition with another model and inserted into theoretical-historical frameworks which relativize its scope, finally turning out to be ambiguous. It is only when Habermas attempts to ground the moral point of view in the structure of reciprocal recognition of subjects acting communicatively, that the legacy of Adorno and Horkheimer will come fully into effect. Interestingly enough, this theoretical elaboration occurs in his reaction to the Kohlberg-Gilligan polemic.

Apart from the gendered aspect of the moral orientations distinguished by Carol Gilligan, Habermas refuses the underlying emotivist dimension of the latter's approach: there is no room for the emotions in the constitution of moral judgment; intuition or moral sentiment, whose reality he does not deny, offer no guarantee that the action it gives rise to is a morally appropriate and justifiable action (Habermas 1991, 195) Furthermore, his interest in Gilligan's studies stems first of all from the fact that his own positions are close to the hypotheses of Lawrence Kohlberg, who defends a moral point of view of the Kantian type. Yet, *by reasoning along the lines of the debate which oppose the latter to Gilligan*, he develops a reformulation of George Herbert Mead's "procedure of ideal role-taking," which, in practical reasoning, allows for a significant taking into account of subjective and contextual particularities. Based on the irreplaceable character of each individual's "yes" or "no," during discussions held not in the privacy of one's mind, but really taking place, this idea has a certain resonance with Joan Tronto's proposition, as encapsulated by her concept of "responsiveness": "Responsiveness suggests a different way to understand the needs of others rather than to put our selves into their position. Instead, it suggests that we consider the other's position as that other expresses it." (Tronto 1993, 136). In addition, Habermas takes the question of the need for a complement to justice in a universalistic morality seriously, which I will come back to in section 2.

Yet, this fragmentary interest is not sufficient in itself to establish real convergence between the two bodies of thought.

First, it may be that in spite of a non feigned sympathy, one always finds oneself in a situation of incompatible grammars, whose meeting, due to different standings in the philosophical field, would, for the ethics of care, take the form of a wrong in the sense Lyotard gives this word, that of an impossibility of receiving acknowledgement for the damage, the loss or even the misinterpretation sustained when taken up by the theories of recognition, in the absence of a theoretical framework and adequate categories. In other words, if one restricts oneself to what the theories of recognition say about care, one may find oneself before an illustration of the spectre raised by Joan Tronto: "perhaps women's morality is just a collection of "moral leftovers," of questions that gain significance only because they are left somewhat open-ended by the commandments and boundaries of public morality [...]. The requirements of justice have traditionally set the boundaries of care" (Tronto 1987, 654)

For Honneth in fact, affective recognition is strictly defined, and cannot be subject to politicization or universalization. While he speaks of universal rights and duties with regard to recognition of the moral autonomy of all human beings, the normativity specific to the forms of recognition associated with care comes with serious restrictions.

On the one hand, "we seem to have duties toward or a special kind of responsibility only for those people with whom we have a specific form of relationship." (Honneth 2005, 44-5) This is without any possible doubt one of the symptoms isolated by Gilligan of the confinement care is subjected to when it is taken up by the ethics of justice: "Within a justice construction, care becomes the mercy that tempers justice, or connotes the special obligations or supererogatory duties that arise in personal relationships" (Gilligan 1995, 36) The result is that this interpretation of care leaves the basic assumptions of a justice framework intact.

On the other hand, it can only be an instance of moral normativity, limited to extreme cases. Because it assumes a state of primordial passivity and receptivity, the intrinsic moral value of the practice of care and the disposition towards it cannot find a systematic place here.

> An obligation to care and to be benevolent can only exist where a person is in a state of such extreme need or hardship that the moral principle of equal treatment can no longer be applied to him or her in a balanced manner. [...] But, conversely, the moment the other person is recognized as an equal being among all others—in that he or she can participate in practical discourses—*the unilateral relation of care must come to an end*; an attitude of benevolence is not permissible toward subjects who are able to articulate their beliefs and views publicly (Honneth, 1995b, 318-9. My emphasis).

This leads us to the second major problem posed by the argument according to which the theories of recognition accommodate themselves to the theoretical constellation of care: that of the emphasis placed on reciprocity, and the regime of equivalence, *i.e.* the possibility of comparison, which underlies the vocabulary of recognition. In fact, as Luc Boltanski has demonstrated, it is "recourse to an equivalent, however basic, which form the basis of the entire theory of reciprocity. In order for the counter-gift to be proportionate in some way to the gift, [...] people must be able to appeal to an instrumentation to link, if only approximately, the actions which compose the sequence." (Boltanski 1990, 174)

In other words, reciprocity is subject to anticipation on the part of each of the partners, who expects from the other an equivalent return (which does not mean identical return, but acceptable in the shared regime of equivalence) to what was given. And there is no doubt that the relationship of recognition is composed of expectations, if not to say measurements.

Moreover, Honneth unambiguously poses the three forms of recognition as "three patterns of reciprocity" (Honneth 1995a, 94), defining the recognition given in the affective sphere as "this symbiotically cherished bond which emerges through mutually desired demarcation." (Honneth 1995a, 107)

It is certain that among the theories of care, there are some which seek to highlight the presence of a form of reciprocity, even in the forms of interaction most hindered by handicap or physical weakness, the cases where the care-receiver is as removed as is possible from the condition of participant involved in a practical discussion favored by Honneth. It is the finality of the numerous reminders in these theories that reciprocity is not symmetry; this is also the principle behind the idea of responsiveness as defended by Tronto, understood as the responsiveness of the care-receiver to the care: "Responsiveness is not the same as reciprocity, but the parallel notion raises some interesting dimensions of responsiveness."[1] (Tronto 1993, 136).

Nonetheless, theories of recognition argue for strong and non tenuous forms of reciprocity. This is what is confirmed, *a contrario*, by the reasoning by which Habermas comes to include animals in our moral community. While Habermas admits the principle of something like a specific responsibility in relation to animals, "a quasi-moral responsibility," this does not take the form of an empathy inspired by beings capable of suffering; it is so because they are partners of interaction, capable of a quasi-reciprocity. "We must be able to ascribe characteristics of agents to animals, among others the ability to initiate utterances and to address them to us" (Habermas 1991, 110). In other words, even in this extreme case, Habermas does not renounce founding practical rationality on reciprocity.

Thus, curbing care whose generalization is perceived as a threat, and assigning an undeniable axiological primacy to reciprocity, the theories of recognition seem to constitute very moderate allies indeed for the ethics of care. Even the publication of *Reification* in 2005 does not question this idea. Admittedly, Honneth now defines "recognition" as a primary form of our relationship to the world that seems to distance his former reluctance:

> our actions do not primarily have the character of an affectively neutral, cognitive stance toward the world, but rather that of an affirmative, existentially coloured style of caring comportment. In living, we constantly concede to the situational circumstances of our world a value of their own, which brings us to be concerned with our relationship to them (Honneth 2008, 38).

Drawing on John Dewey's idea of practical involvement, Lukács's engaged practice and Cavell's notion of acknowledgement, he refers to a fundamental non-cognitive stance towards things and persons such as we experience situations in such a way that we "take care" to maintain a fluent interaction with our surroundings. Yet, this book speaks of a more fundamental level of recognition than that addressed in his previous studies, which are in no way called into question. This primary form of recognition "is not intended to contain any norms of positive concern or respect. Nor does it claim that certain positive, benevolent feelings are at work" (Honneth 2008, 151), as Honneth repeats in his response to his commentators, including Judith Butler and Martin Jay. Love and hate, ambivalence and coldness, can all be expressions of this primary recognition. But at the higher level, where there the three spheres of recognition described above are distinguished and which involves taking over the other's perspective, hate, ambivalence and coldness may in turn be seen as denials of recognition. In other words, this idea of primordial recognition is probably closer to the notion of empathy than care, such as defined by theorists of care.

Perhaps it is necessary then to retrace our steps and pursue the reasoning on a deeper level. From this point of view, the place attributed by the defenders of care to the solicitude due to the other in his vulnerability, his intrinsic dependence and needs, their insistence on the awareness of the harm that can be inflicted upon him and on the notion of responsibility, seem to provide a promising starting point.

For I believe it is possible to demonstrate that the notion of vulnerability is central to theories of recognition, insofar as they refer to, often with the intention of reformulating Hegel's struggle for recognition, George Herbert Mead's work, *Mind, Self and Society from the Standpoint of a Social Behaviorist*, according to which consciousness, "far from being a precondition to the social act [...], is preconditioned by this very act." (Mead 1934, 16). From this point of view, my reasoning here goes further than the theorists of recognition who are the heirs to Critical Theory to include all contemporary thinkers who approach the problematic from these premises of Hegelian inspiration.

## 2. Topography of the idea of constitutional vulnerability

Following Mead, for Charles Taylor, Jürgen Habermas, Ernst Tugendhat and Axel Honneth among others, the self can only develop in a process of interaction: when a self does appear, it always involves an experience of another. They consider the formation of identity as dependent on multiple recognitions or misrecognitions. Habermas, for example, argues that individuation occurs in socialization and that interlocutors are also subjects who face each other with a claim to be recognized as irreplaceable individuals. Charles Taylor, for his part, returns to Mead's idea of others as "significant others" and claims State protections for "distinct societies" as networks of interlocution in which the intersubjective constitution of self occurs. (Taylor 1994, 50)

Accordingly individuality is constituted both through intersubjective recognition and through one's self-understanding as mediated by intersubjectivity. Hence the need for the other's recognition experienced by each of us, and our *vulnerability* to its possible denial.

Let me compare this with earlier uses of the idea of recognition. What motivates the struggle or the claim for recognition in contemporary theories of recognition is not the Hegelian *desire* of the absolute self. According to the interpretation of the *Phenomonelogy of Spirit* proposed by Alexandre Kojève, the human begins at the point where man's "biological desire to preserve his life" is subordinated to "his human desire for Recognition." "Human desire, therefore, must win out over this desire of preservation. In other words, man's humanity 'comes to light' only if he risks his [animal] life for the sake of his human Desire" (Kojève 1980, 7). It is this desire of recognition—and not a *need*—that initiates the life and death struggle. Even earlier, in Rousseau, what motivates the struggle or the claim for recognition is an insurmountable desire for approval. Such is the conclusion to the *Discourse on the Origin of Inequality*: "The savage lives in himself, the sociable man always outside of himself knows how to live only in the opinion of others, and it is, so to speak, from their judgment alone that he draws the sentiment of his own existence." (Rousseau 1996, 193) In other words, as Tzvetan Torodov puts it, Rousseau makes the desire for prestige and glory "the threshold beyond which one can speak of humankind." (Todorov, 1995, 56)

In clear opposition to these earlier occurrences, for Charles Taylor, for instance, "non-recognition or misrecognition ... can be a form of oppression, imprisoning someone in a false, distorted, reduced mode of being. Beyond simple lack of respect, it can inflict a grievous wound, saddling people with crippling self-hatred. Due recognition is not just a courtesy *but a vital human need*." (Taylor 1994, 25. My emphasis) In Axel Honneth's words, "because the normative self-image of each and every individual human being ... is dependant on the possibility of being continually backed up by others, the experience of being disrespected carries with it the danger of an injury that can bring the identity of the person as a whole to the point of collapse." (Honneth 1995a, 131-132)

Strikingly enough, the word "vulnerability" appears only rarely in these theories, especially in Honneth's earlier works. It has only been recently and intermittently that he has made use of the word, qualifying it as moral. Stating that the first step in developing a morality of recognition consists in the essential proof that the possibility of moral injuries follows from the intersubjectivity of the human life form, he wrote that "Human beings are vulnerable in the specific manner we call « moral » because they owe their identity to the construction of a practical self-relation that is, from the beginning, dependent upon the help and affirmation of other human beings." (Honneth 2005, 51)

It is, perhaps surprisingly, Jürgen Habermas who links his theory of recognition to an anthropology of vulnerability in a way that is both the most asserted and the most repeated, speaking of "extreme vulnerability" as a central aspect of discourse ethics: "Unless the subject externalizes in interpersonal relations through language, he is unable to form that inner center that is his personal identity. This explains the almost constitutional insecurity and chronic fragility of personal identity—an insecurity that is antecedent to cruder threats to the integrity of life and limb." (Habermas 1995, 199)

More specifically, at the core of struggles for recognition is the idea that not being recognized means being unable to maintain a *practical* relation-to-self. Thus, the idea of constitutional vulnerability has led current theories of recognition to reformulate normative concepts like autonomy in terms of this new ontology of the individual.

Autonomy is in fact *conditional on* intersubjective consideration. While in the liberal tradition autonomy is ensured by guaranteeing rights, in theories of recognition the relation between rights and autonomy is indirect. The existence of rights only provides the necessary conditions for self-respect, and it is from self-respect that autonomy will (eventually) grow. In other words, these theories take into consideration the fact that agency is endangered when the individual is not capable of nurturing the conviction that his aspirations are worth pursuing. Here empirical and normative elements converge, since, while it can certainly be possible to act autonomously in spite of practices and institutions that perpetually express depreciation, it is not fair that some people have to bear this weight to attain autonomy. (Honneth/Anderson 2005) Far from referring to the absence of restrictions, autonomy is in this way made dependent on a context of social relations capable of bringing about the feeling of one's ability and legitimacy to act.

The idea of public autonomy, the collective and deliberative process of society's self-government or self-determination, is affected by the same reasoning. Free access to contexts of communication and mutual recognition in which people can acquire and consolidate their identity, articulate their understanding of themselves, and develop their own life plans also guarantees their development as autonomous *citizens*, since, as Kymlicka puts it, "it is only through having access to a societal culture that people have access to a range of meaningful options." (Kymlicka 1994, 83) That is why the politics of identity formulated by Charles Taylor defends the subordination of moral and public autonomy to the health of collective identities, based on an assumed equivalence between recognition of my group and recognition of myself. When the problematic of recognition doesn't bring about a reformulation of the experience of injustice in the language of *collective* identities, one can also consider that individuals' capacity for action is threatened when they are not in a position to believe that their aspirations are worth pursuing, owing to institutionalized patterns of cultural value that disparage their distinctive characteristics or those assigned to them. (Honneth, Anderson 2005) It then can be argued that being unable to assert their claims and aspirations, they are denied the status of legitimate co-legislators.

Here, the rupture with the perspective of a subject only considered fully as such when attesting to his sovereignty over himself constitutes a premise that is wholly shared with theories of care. As Carol

Gilligan writes, "as a framework for moral decision, care is grounded in the assumption that self and other are interdependent, an assumption reflected in a view of action as responsive and, therefore, as arising in relationship rather than the view of action as emanating from within the self, and therefore self-governed" (Gilligan 1995, 36)

It also follows with this type of premise that Hegelian theories of recognition place us before the fact of selves always being available for harming, recalling man's physical vulnerability—the fact of bodies always being available for wounding.

Jean-Marc Ferry notes that "vulnerability is perhaps the notion which best correlates the idea of an infringement-not-to-be-made-to-the integrity of X." (Ferry 1991, 121) And as it happens, in both bodies of theories one finds the same form of vulnerability defined by the likelihood of infringement, and the idea deduced from it of an ethical attitude which consists in hesitating before the perspective of the damage which we could inflict: "In the end, choice hinges on the determination of "where the greater responsibility lies," a determination based on an assessment of vulnerability, a relative estimate of who will be more hurt" (Gilligan 1982, 42).

We must now draw out the precise moral implications of the constitutional vulnerability assumed by contemporary theories of recognition in order to determine to what extent the homology with the ethics of care applies.

## 3. The moral implications of a constitutional vulnerability

Vulnerability implies more than susceptibility to certain sorts of harm; it implies that harm is avoidable. Hence the possibility of advocating an obligation to protect the vulnerable, an obligation to prevent harm from occurring.

Insofar as Honneth's theory relies on the idea of deeply rooted *expectations* of recognition directed toward multiple others, who consequently bear the burden of recognition, it assumes such an obligation. "Built into the structure of human interaction there is a normative expectation that one will meet with recognition of others, or at least an implicit assumption that one will be given positive consideration in the plans of others" (Honneth 1995a, 44).

However what then is the nature of the moral attitude which consists in responding to this expectation, or, to put it differently, of the attitude which causes one to hesitate before the perspective of the wound we might inflict?

According to John Wilson, in the case of a relationship of dependence, A's concern for B's *good* (here B's personal integrity) entitles A to intervene only if the relevant aspect of B's good is A's business, and this requires that at least one of the following obtains: (1) A has a responsibility toward B which extends to that aspect of his good; (2) A has a legitimate interest in that aspect of B's good. (Wilson 1977, 312)

Considered closely, both aspects can be found in the problematic of recognition.

Honneth recently attempted to establish the systematic relationship between morality and recognition, starting from the idea that "if it is correct to say that the core of moral injuries is located in the refusal of recognition, then that suggests, inversely, that moral attitudes are connected with the exercise of recognition" (Honneth 2005, 50). Morality is then assigned the purpose of protecting against the dangers referred to. The moral point of view is then not doubled by a corrective principle granting expectations of recognition, rather it finds itself redefined as made up of various attitudes "we have to adopt to protect human beings from injuries" (Honneth 2005, 51). It has to encompass not just moral respect, but *three* independent modes of recognition, including solidarity and this kind of recognition, "which has the character of affective concern, such as care or love" (Honneth 2005, 52). Responding to an expectation of recognition thus stems more from moral obligations articulated to norms than from a responsibility, norms deriving their binding force from the validity of norms of interaction that claim to rest on good reasons.

Nonetheless, the circle of persons **supposed to** assume such moral attitudes varies from one mode of recognition to the next, and the moral attitudes borne by each mode are likely to enter into conflict

(Honneth 2005, 54). For these reasons, the distinction between the moral obligation borne by the morality depicted by Honneth and the idea of individual or a collective "special responsibility," entailed by the peculiar vulnerability of someone else to our actions and choices, advocated by Robert Goodin in his book *Protecting the Vulnerable* (Goodin 1985, 205) is not as solid as seems at first glance, at least not as solid as claimed by Gilligan. According to her in fact, in the perspective of the ethics of care, the

> moral problem arises from conflicting responsibilities rather than from competing rights and requires for its resolution a mode of thinking that is contextual and narrative rather than formal and abstract. This conception of morality as concerned with the activity of care centers moral development around the understanding of *responsibility* and relationships, just as the conception of morality as fairness ties moral development to the understanding of rights and *rules*" (Gilligan 1982, 19. My emphasis).

In Honneth's theory, as in Goodin's model, the moral claim is a claim upon me because, and only if, the other is vulnerable to my actions. In other words, the response is called for as much by norms as by the relationship itself. Honneth strikingly underlines for instance the moral relevance of the relationship for the sphere of affective recognition: "Through our acts of affection, we encourage another person to open himself or herself to us emotionally in such a way that he or she is rendered so vulnerable as to deserve, instead of mere respect, all the benevolence we can muster" (Honneth 2007b, 178).

Habermas similarly sees morality as compensating for the extreme vulnerability of subjects who become individualized in socialization, by providing forms of reciprocal recognition, however the arrangement is singularly different. Human fragility is endowed with a specific ethical force, calling for the suspension of the exercise of a power to infringe deeply, for its non-usage, a call which resonates in our moral intuitions.

Correlatively, Habermas assigns morality with a double task: that of conveying individuals' inviolability by demanding the equal respect of each and every person's dignity; that of protecting the intersubjective relations of reciprocal recognition through which individuals maintain **themselves** as members of a community. These two complementary demands correspond to the principles of justice and solidarity. Whereas one postulates equal respect and equality of rights for each individual, the other demands empathy and assistance for the well-being of one's neighbor. And Habermas dismisses the specter of a relegation of solidarity to lesser and anecdotal forms, the possibility of the Lyotardian wrong which I mentioned earlier, by stating clearly: "Justice conceived deontologically requires solidarity as its reverse side. It is a question not so much of two moments that supplement each other as of two aspects of the same thing" (Habermas 1990, 244).

It will then appear that while he admits to the need for a complement to justice—doing so, let us not forget, in reaction to the Gilligan-Kohlberg debate—he carefully avoids giving it the name of care. Yet, unlike Honneth, he does not hesitate to use the word responsibility; solidarity "is rooted in the realization that each person must take *responsibility for the other* because as consociates all must have in interest in the integrity of their shared life context in the same way" (Habermas 1990, 242. My emphasis).

However with this last quotation, there has already been a shift towards the other possible origin of the ethical attitude in the framework of a relationship of dependence proposed by Wilson (A has a legitimate interest in that aspect of B's good); it is with the latter that the deep-rooted, architectonic similarity with the theories of care re-emerges.

Inasmuch as the idea of vulnerability inherent in theories of recognition is that of a shared vulnerability—we are all creatures individuated only through socialization, we are all vulnerable and in need of consideration—recognition is also frequently formulated according to Wilson's second kind of legitimate concern, as relying on a *mutual need*, as opposed to a *mutual duty*. In other words, each of us has a legitimate interest in recognition of the others. As Mead puts it, "it is that self which is able to maintain itself in the community, that is recognized in the community in so far as it recognizes the others." (Mead 1934, 196) Honneth gives this idea a much more existential twist: "In order to be able to offer a stranger recognition associated with concern (based on solidarity), for his or her way of life, I need to have already had the shock of an experience that taught me that we share, in an existential sense, our exposure to certain dangers." (Honneth 1995a, 90)

In such a perspective, recognition is motivated neither by obedience to duty, nor by benevolent spontaneity. The good of the other is the medium to achieve my own good. Here there emerges the perspective of a vulnerability that is both ineradicable—the condition of possibility of my existence— and for this very reason, carrying the need to protect that of others—the foundation of my moral attitude before others. In other words, one finds oneself here before a variant of the reasoning developed by Eva Feder Kittay, when she asserts, regarding the relationship of dependence, that a subject who "refuses to support this bond absolves itself from its most fundamental obligation—its obligation to its founding possibility." (1998, 131) As Kelly Oliver puts it in a book which is moreover a critical reading of Hegelian theories of recognition: "Response-ability is the founding possibility of subjectivity and its most fundamental obligation." (Oliver 2001, 91)

Beyond formal references, it is therefore because of an underlying anthropology of vulnerability that contemporary theories of recognition—which present human beings as constitutively fragile and exposed—overlap with certain preoccupations and formulations of the ethics of care. It enables them in particular to defend a reflection on the nature and the finality of the moral attitude whose arguments are constructed in a way that is similar to what is found among the defenders of care.

The fact remains that while the theory of recognition allows to conceptualize "the infringement not to be made" without any problem, it does not manage, at least in its current developments, to project the image of what a given or successful recognition would be, or a recognition granted to a subjectivity already adversely affected or maimed, or to define a response to a normative expectation which is not limited to an abstention. This is what is also highlighted by the confrontation with the ethics of care, a confrontation which enables to distinguish two interlocked[2] vulnerabilities. This shared vulnerability, which we cannot renounce without ceasing to be human, this "enabling vulnerability," to borrow an expression created by Judith Butler in a radically different context (Butler 1996, 2), which I have been principally preoccupied with up to this point, is articulated to a strong, "extensive vulnerability" (Kittay 1999, 65), limited to some people or identifiable states of our life history, which is no longer a potential but a materialized vulnerability, and which calls for more than for a negatively defined attitude, in other words, which calls for care in the fullest sense of the term.

Inversely, theories of recognition invite us to envision a demand for the preservation of personal integrity in similar terms to the preservation of physical integrity, which, since Hobbes at least, has been presented as the primary function of political institutions. Theories of recognition thus seem to argue that we need to broaden the concept of justice. It becomes necessary to envisage integrating within it, alongside a fundamental right to physical integrity, a right that is just as fundamental to satisfying the conditions for a positive relationship to self. Without this right to personal integrity, the agent is incapable of valorizing his own existence and forming a life project likely to give a positive content to the negative freedom which the classical formal rights protect.

Now, such a conception of justice would not, *a priori*, enable us to carry out a rational deduction of the institutions required for a perfectly just society, like the deduction Rawls sought to make in his *Theory of Justice*. This concept of justice would be a tool of social criticism, justifying the legitimacy of social transformations to reduce misrecognitions within a real society· The political task would then consist in a pragmatic critique of institutions so as to tend towards the elimination of every denial of recognition or misrecognition through progressive and experimental adjustments. (Honneth 1995a, 179) The unfinished aspect of a social and moral theory first defined negatively, in reference to moral or mental wounds likely to be inflicted, is also what enables its relatively easy transposition to the political field, by opening up the perspective of a succession of struggles and of a fragmentary elucidation of the normative content of recognition.

## Notes

[1] Similarly, Andries Baart underlined during the conference that he preferred to speak of care-seekers rather than care-receivers.

[2] I would like to thank Christa Schnabl for having drawn my attention to this point.

# 11.
# *Humane dignity*

Margaret Urban Walker

Dignity is a majestic and powerful idea not only in modern and contemporary ethics, but in contemporary political discourse as well. References to dignity are common in moral philosophy, being part of a relatively tight circle of ideas that includes rational agency, autonomous choice, humanity, respect, rights, recognition, decency, and moral worth. The idea did not originate with Kant, but Kant put, it seems, a definitive and lasting stamp upon it and the circle of moral ideas to which it belongs. This is not to say that dignity is tightly and uniformly interdefined with these other notions in one particular way. The least varying connection, however, is that dignity is a kind of moral worth human beings possess that entitles them to respect. This, with variations, is the kind of thing moral philosophers and some political theorists say. People who are not moral philosophers, but who command the concept of dignity, may say that some treatment of a person is "beneath" his or her dignity, that it is indecent or disrespectful to treat a person that way; they may even say that someone's dignity was lost or destroyed. We also, in common speech, have the idea of an "indignity," a treatment beneath or out of keeping with what a human being deserves and one a human being should not, as we say, "suffer."

One reason more and more people, in many places in the world, do command this concept with some of its standard connections is the global spread of human rights discourse. From the adoption of the United Nations Universal Declaration of Human Rights, with its opening pronouncement that all members of the human family possess "inherent dignity," and "all human beings are born free and equal in dignity and right," the discourse of human rights and its allied language of dignity is a twenty-first century lingua franca of politics in what is called the "world community," circulating the concept of dignity world-wide. I do not mean to say that it is only due to the European tradition that gave form to the legal and moral regime of human rights that human beings have some notion of a particular kind of human worth. On the contrary, I suppose instead that there is something in the concept of dignity recognizable to people of many regions, cultures, and faiths that has enabled this idea to be grasped and affirmed as widely as it has been, given the circulation of human rights discourse (on the argument about the Western European nature of human rights, see Sen 1999; Lauren 2003; and Afshari 2007). In our time a body of ostensibly authoritative declarations and conventions invoke the idea of dignity as a fundamental–indeed foundational–premise from which an impressive assortment of human rights of several types are claimed to flow.

I want to re-examine the idea of dignity, starting with what is problematic in an understanding of dignity that connects it in a tight circle with full or fully mature capacity for moral agency, essentially an idealized and exclusive concept of dignity for which Kant's thinking, especially in his *Groundwork of the metaphysic of morals*, is the paradigm. I want to discuss some strategies, overlapping and mutually compatible but distinct, for reconstructing this concept in a more humane and humanly inclusive way. The three "humanizing" strategies I will suggest in conclusion are naturalizing dignity, rendering dignity relationally, and differentiating our concept of dignity. These strategies are intended to preserve the normative force of the concept of dignity as an ideal of human interaction, recognition, and concern; they continue to give a central place in our understanding of dignity to those who are fully, symmetrically, and reciprocally accountable to each other. But they attempt to widen the net which catches the humanity of many who may not appear to be the paradigm cases of full, symmetrical and reciprocal accountability.

To begin, I want to look at the nexus of notions with which dignity is intertwined in the Kantian formation, to see what is problematic about the circle they form, and to consider some alternatives to reconstructing the concept in the ways I will explore. I then turn to these strategies of reconstruction, to invite a conversation about what is promising or worrisome in these ways of rethinking dignity, or whether there are other ways, and to invite consideration in thinking about why we need a concept of dignity at all, and what moral work we need the idea of dignity to do.

## 1. Worries about the "Kantian" idea of dignity

An ideal of dignity deeply rooted in the Kantian tradition is both idealized and multiply exclusive: beings with rational wills and hence powers of autonomous choice have that distinctive moral value called 'dignity.' All such beings possess dignity, but *only* such beings do, and dignity refers to the *only* value there is that is moral value. All and only such beings deserve respect, the paradigm moral attitude, for this view. The feature that qualifies such beings is their endowment with rational will and thus autonomous choice, and that feature is also that about them which we must aim to respect, even if it can be argued that we must refrain from, for example, physically damaging or avoidable painful physical and psychological treatment as a way to show respect to the rational will "within."

This conception of dignity and its implications for moral attitude and behavior is multiply exclusive. Those human beings who do not possess rational wills and the power of autonomous choice do not possess the all-important moral value of dignity. Since there is no other kind of value that is moral value, it seems that beings, including human beings, who do not possess the entitling capacity not only fail to possess dignity and to be entitled to respect, they seem to fail to possess any distinct moral value. They may nonetheless possess "relative" value due to their importance to others who happen to love and cherish them, but it seems they are not entitled to the responses or attitudes constitutive of truly moral recognition. At the same time, the responses of love, delight, cherishing, care, pity, and concern these human beings evoke in others are not seen as forms of truly moral recognition. In the case of those who do possess rational will and so dignity, on this view, what we must morally respond to in them is the feature by virtue of which they possess that moral value, their capacity for rational willing, not their ability to suffer pain or humiliation or rejection, for example, unless these forms of treatment can be shown to at the same time also affront their status and function as autonomous beings or perhaps to interfere with means necessary to act so as to treat persons as ends. Furthermore, what the dignity of these fully operational moral agents commands on the part of others of the same moral status is respect as autonomous beings, but only this. Other "feelings," such as compassion, sympathy, empathy, pity, admiration, or gratitude, are merely "pathological" on the Kantian scheme; feelings that are mere animal inclinations can endow their objects with a value relative to human desires, but this relative value is not moral value.

I don't suppose that many contemporary neo-Kantians, or even contemporary Kantians, are willing to defend this view in precisely this stark form, but I think the original Kantian logic is likely to follow the notion of dignity in at least this way: Dignity will be associated with moral capacity, moral capacity will be associated with a rather high level and sophisticated kind of rational deliberation and choice, the possession of the relevant endowments for moral agency will confer an entitlement to respectful treatment, and respectful treatment will be that which acknowledges and perhaps affirms the value of just this sophisticated moral capacity. Explicating Kant in a way that endorses his view, Christine Korsgaard says that "the distinctive nature of humanity *as such*, is simply the capacity to take a rational interest in something," and "humanity is the power of rational choice, but only when choice is fully rational is humanity fully realized" (Korsgaard 1996, 114, 123). Insofar as humanity functions positively in our moral valuation, "It is your powers as an agent that are to be promoted" (127). Axel Honneth, in his insightful account of recognition, identifies as a common premise of modern moral thinking (shared, for example, by Hegel and Mead) that "subjects are to be recognized as both autonomous and individualized beings," both equal and particular (Honneth 1995, 171, 175). The addition of particularity is important, and I affirm it later, although the standing in question envisions a morally fully-fledged and morally responsible agent. In Stephen Darwall's recent book, *The Second Person Standpoint*, dignity is "the status of an equal member of the moral community" to hold others who are such accountable; the second-person standpoint defines the moral community, and second-personal address presupposes "a common normative standing as free and rational persons" (Darwall 2006, 243, 265). Darwall also says that "any second-personal address seeks reciprocal recognition by its very nature" (265), apparently equating reciprocal recognition (two-way recognition with parties aware of its mutual character), with symmetrical recognition (reciprocal recognition *as equal*), an equation that I will believe must be questioned. I mention these views in lieu of a survey to suggest that the tight links among dignity, moral agency, moral worth, respect, and recognition, and the categorical (all or nothing) logic of these concepts, stemming from the Kantian paradigm, are continuing and forceful.

The tight circle of concepts to which dignity has belonged produces exclusions, and these exclusions follow from not only the original Kantian but also prevalent neo-Kantian ideas about dignity as the paradigmatic, or the only, moral standing and its links to full moral agency. They unavoidably raise questions: What of human beings who do not possess full moral capacity (even defined by a threshold of ability) or who possess a limited or reduced kind of it? What of those forms of pain, suffering, insult or diminishment that human beings endure at the hands of others which either do not directly assault their moral capacity, or that not only assault or insult moral capacity but which punish, hurt, refuse, or repudiate what is human in them that is not, or not only, their moral capacity? If respect is the paradigm attitude that salutes another's moral value, what then of those other attitudes that grasp and address another's humanity, like compassion, cherishing, pity, and gratitude? And what of the uniquely human features of individual expression, attachment, desire, joy, sadness, and grief that embody the individuality of human individuals who possess less or little in the way of those rational capacities, or whose capacities are differently configured?

## 2. Do we need the concept of dignity, and why?

Perhaps the concept of dignity is part of a metaphysical mythology we do not need, and one that stands in the way of addressing well-being and ill treatment and so the comfort and suffering of human beings, and perhaps other beings, in a realistic and humane fashion. Such a view is at home with some kinds of utilitarian thinking. In one recent op-ed piece Singer applies philosophical views for which he is already well-known. Writing on the case of Ashley, a 9-year-old child whose severe mental disabilities give her the functioning of a 3-month-old, Singer responds to critics of her parents' decision to treat her chemically and surgically to keep her small and light in size and sexually nonmature in order to better care for her. Singer criticizes a statement by Ashley's parents that this treatment will give her more dignity. Singer's response is that dignity is an irrelevant category to apply to any individual with human's 3-month-old mental capacity, however precious Ashley is to her parents and siblings. Singer says, "what matters in Ashley's life is that she should not suffer" (Singer 2007). This viewpoint challenges those who consider dignity important in this case to explain how dignity can even make sense in this case, and in many other cases of several reduced mental capacity.

Soran Reader has laid down another aggressive challenge, as it were from the opposite end, to what she terms the "agential bias" that permeates American and European moral philosophy in the self-portrait of persons as paradigmatically "active, capable, free, and independent" (Reader 2007, 603-604). Reader argues that the other, non-agential aspects of a person–suffering, weakness, vulnerability, constraint, dependency–are elements of human life that should receive attention for the profound degree to which they shape our lives. More strongly, they are not fallings away or privations or lapses in being a person, but are in fact presupposed, according to her, to our more highly valued agential features (588). If that is so, we should "recognize and dignify" the non-agential aspects as just as much aspects of "full, complex personhood" (592). Reader lays down a challenge to incorporate (an appropriately loaded word, with its reference to our essentially embodied existence) many more aspects of what is human into a picture of humanity and (I assume) its dignity, but also to abandon the idea that certain moral capacities, especially forms of intellectual capacity and executive control, have a preeminent place, even if they still have an important one.

I hasten to apologize to Singer, and even more so to Reader (who does not address the topic of dignity directly), for not engaging these important views in depth. I use their views here purely to exemplify some striking challenges to the usefulness–the scope and sufficiency–of the concept of dignity predicated on the idea of certain higher moral and mental capacities. They focus questions sharply about the extent to which a picture of human beings as uniquely endowed with moral personality, a valuation of human beings to the extent that they do possess that endowment, and a definition of that endowment largely in terms of normal adult human intellectual and reflective capacities and capacities of independent self-control, intellectual or not, adequately captures the moral value of humanity or those features which determine the moral pull of one human being on another. These challenges have the virtue of raising a stark question: is it a *moral mistake* to be drawn into a way of thinking that treats the full complement and development of mature moral capacities as an endowment of human beings that lays special claims upon us in our treatments of and responses to them?

In response, I take the position that it is not a mistake, and it is a necessity to acknowledge that full moral capacity–the capacity to engage at a threshold level in relations of reciprocal accountability organized by normative expectations that assume the authority of moral and other norms–is a distinctive feature of human beings with distinct moral significance (see Walker 2006 on the central role of accountability and trust in sustaining moral relations). I do not disagree with Reader that there is an agential bias in our dominant philosophical conception of human persons, but I do not think the moral weight that attaches to agency is simply a mistake. We wouldn't have morality as we know it without this *characteristic, although not universal*, set of human capacities. All those who possess some functional threshold level of this capacity are indeed placed distinctly with respect to all others who possess it: they are bound to participation in fully mutual and symmetrical accountability, the calling-to-account of one another without which no norms have effective social authority. There is no need to deny that a normal and fully reflective mature ability to participate in interpersonal accounting is a distinctive human species characteristic that makes possible the exquisitely intricate normative structure of shared human life of which morality is one part. There is increasing scientific evidence that this capacity is not entirely cognitive, but involves emotional sensitivities as well, and surely more attention must be paid to the embodied character of the expression, recognition, and responsiveness of human beings in ways that constitute moral relations.

On the one hand, a view such as Reader's is too quick to diminish the moral significance of the difference that human agential capacities make to there being such a dimension of human life as morality. On the other hand, it minimizes differences between those vulnerabilities, dependencies, and passivities that are woven through, or that predictably punctuate, uncompromised human agency and those that are in fact disabling of agency in some respect. Disability theorists teach us to be very careful how we conceive of features of individuals as disabling when forms of disablement really arise from the hostility of humanly constructed physical and social environments to the expression of some people's agency (Wendell 1996; Scully 2009). Still, there are disabilities that transcend the limits of environmental hospitality and diminish or circumscribe agency. The ethics of care and dependency teach us to remember that we all always vulnerable and interdependent, and that all of us at some times in our lives are among those not fully able (Tronto 1993; Sevenhuijsen 1998; Kittay 1999). These facts and our universally shared experiences of them, whether they are admitted and emphasized or not, are as integral to humanity as are capacities for self-control, reflective choice, reciprocal understandings and interpersonal accountability.

To say that all those who possess some functional threshold level of this capacity can distinctively enter into fully symmetrical accountability, however, is not to say that *only* those who can participate in fully symmetrical reciprocity with each other are parties to the practices of responsibility of which accountability is always a central dimension. First, there are many reciprocal relations of accountability that are not fully symmetrical. Institutional roles of authority and subordination between those equally capable provide one example. Relations between children and adults, not equally capable in all or many respects, and more generally relations between those lacking certain competencies and those who possess them, relations of care or guardianship, are others. Many of these relations involve forms of non-symmetrical reciprocity: they are relations in which there are normatively acceptable ways for the participants to respond to each other, but their respective prerogatives and obligations with respect to each other are not identical. Many forms of these nonsymmetrical but reciprocal relations are morally defensible, and even morally required. Yet it is also true that historically the model of morally justified asymmetrical relations has repeatedly been used to justify arbitrary and socially imposed asymmetries on adults fully capable of and entitled to symmetrical standings: men over women; the aristocrat over the commoner; higher over lower class or caste; civilized over barbarian; free over slave, etc. (Aristotle's ethical and political views are the classic philosophical loci of this kind of philosophical apology for hierarchy, but the patterns of thinking has persisted down the centuries.) Furthermore, all differentials in reciprocal moral standing, whether justified or not, are subject to abuse. The different or unequal bases of reciprocity may be exaggerated, improperly generalized over areas where they need not obtain, or simply exploited by the stronger to exercise power over those who are unlikely to be able to complain, or whose complaints are unlikely to be credited. But the indefensibility of some forms of nonsymmetrical reciprocity does not erase the reality and defensibility of other unavoidable kinds of nonsymmetrical, yet reciprocal, relations.

Further, the competence to participate, wholesale or retail, in relations of reciprocal accountability does not exhaust what is valuable to or among human beings. This competence is not the only thing about human beings that we reasonably cherish and seek to protect, enjoy, and enhance through practices of responsibility that embody moral values. Human beings lacking in forms of competence to participate in moral accounting need not be lacking in other valuable and valued features of humanity, for only some of these valued human features require capacities for reflective choice or responsible agency. Other such features cherished by and among human beings are humanly distinctive forms of attention, orientation to our surroundings, expression, feeling, connection, and relation. Peter Singer is impatient with the idea that a child, especially an infant, can be said to have dignity. But this is a real question: how might we apply that idea to the infant and the child? It is obvious that young children can experience shaming and degrading conditions of belittlement, dirtiness, poverty, or abuse, but it is also true that even small children have cognitive capacities and emotional differentiation that infants do not. And yet, despite Singer's impatience, people very commonly say they believe severely mentally compromised human beings, despite a lack of certain cognitive and emotional functioning, should nonetheless be treated, as much as is practically possible, with dignity. The challenge is to rebut Singer's presumption that this is a sentimental rhetoric. Rebutting this presumption, though, might involve precisely, among other things, attending to the role of certain sentiments that are understood when expressed, perceived, or responded to as signature attributes of the human kind, and hence ones that figure in what we are able to think of as an adequately dignified or undignified situation or treatment for a human being.

Dignity need not be the only morally weighty consideration pertaining to the treatment of human beings. One might worry about trying to pack too much into the idea of dignity, or making too much of our moral sensibility rest upon considerations of dignity. This itself might be a symptom of domination by a Kantian (or more broadly, an agential) perspective in which dignity monopolizes the moral field. After all, on the face of it, suffering and well-being have their own moral weight as considerations about how to treat human beings as well as other non-human creatures. On the other hand, over a wide range of cases, one does not grasp what human beings can suffer or what it means for them to fare well without understanding particular forms of suffering that arise from human sensibilities and particular forms of enjoyment that are imbued with humanly distinctive desires and responses, again not confined to rational agency. Importantly, it is unmistakably human as well to experience particular forms of suffering and delight at the distinctively human experiences of *other* human beings, including others' experience of our own reactions to them. It is unmistakably human to experience indignation and pity at the treatment of others, and also to react emotionally to the reactions or failures to react of those among us who witness pitiable, degrading, or unconscionable treatment of others, whether or not those so badly treated are capable of sharing or appreciating these reactions. It does not seem forced to think of human dignity as implicated in these reactions to human beings (nor does it require us, for example, to deny that there might be analogous reactions to the treatment of other feeling beings). As was stressed by theorists such as David Hume and Adam Smith in the sentimentalist moral tradition (Kant's contemporary counterpoint), morality has greatly to do with capacities for "fellow feeling" of both positive and negative sorts, and with feelings about the feelings that we show and that are shown by others. Perhaps dignity has more to do with the recognition and the operations of this aspect of our common humanity than has yet been fully explored.

How might we begin to rethink the idea of dignity to capture some of this complexity? We need, I believe, to preserve the truth that human beings as a species-type possess special features in virtue of which they are capable of constituting moral relations, and that all human beings capable of reciprocal and symmetrical accountability do stand in a special relation to each other as bearers of full and symmetrical mutual accountability. Yet other human beings are encompassed in relations of reciprocity that are not entirely or fully symmetrical, and some are held among us in a kind of trust in and for humanity even if they are capable of little or very partial reciprocity. Finally, there is much that is distinctively (whether or not uniquely) human that we have reason to value among ourselves (and not only for the reason that it distinguishes us as human). The question remains: how is the tight circle of notions connected to dignity opened to constitute an arc of recognition, reciprocity, responsibility, and response that fully comprehends (in both senses of that term—to include and to understand) humanity?

## 3. Humanizing dignity

I begin from the idea that dignity is a *standing*, that is, a socially and interpersonally effective position comprising values, prerogatives, entitlements, liabilities or responsibilities that others are bound to recognize and in response to which others and the one who possesses dignity act and interact. We might think of dignity as realized in the shared understanding and coordinated expression of this standing by ones who possess it and others with respect to them. If dignity is a standing in this way, and so is an essentially interpersonal construction, then dignity is underpinned and required, but not fully determined, by independent features of the one who possesses it. To possess dignity is to be able to express and exercise this standing, at least to some extent and in some ways, and the expression and exercise require that others not block or thwart this expression and exercise, but also to have others give at least implicit recognition and in some degree appropriate supporting responses to its expression and exercise. Dignity then is constituted in a successful enactment of at least some of its characteristic exercises both by one who possesses dignity and those who must recognize it. The possessor of dignity must exercise capacities and engage in expressions that exemplify and claim dignity, and those who must give it recognition must also exercise their capacities to provide confirming and supporting responses. If there are multiple capacities and expressions from either side that exhibit and affirm humanity, then those characteristic exercises and responses that constitute dignity will be multiple. It will not be only the display and recognition of some rational capacities that will claim or affirm the dignity of human beings.

The way I have just described it makes dignity an interpersonally effective standing that is multiply conditioned or relative. It is interpersonal, and so requires uptake to be successfully expressed. Its enactment is also relative to certain capacities relevant to its exercise; if there is not only one human capacity that grounds dignity, then it can be expressed and can seek recognition through some capacities rather than others, either at a particular time or over time. Finally, its successful enactment requires a certain threshold that is recognizably human, whether or not it is paradigmatic for the fullest development of a particular kind of human functioning; since uptake is a crucial part of successful expression, others must be able to respond in particular ways that affirm and complement its recognizable humanness. I hasten to acknowledge that this is all abstract in the extreme. I quickly turn to three directions in which we might seek concretely to rethink dignity as an interpersonally effective standing: *naturalizing* it; rendering it explicitly *relational*; and *differentiating* it in terms of multiple morally affirming (and rejecting) responses.

### *Naturalizing dignity*

To decisively break from the abiding Kantian tendency to tie dignity solely to some form of rational capacity requires thinking about what *in* humans as we *actually* find them we *as* humans recognize as deeply human, and so what it is we have reason to value in valuing human beings. I have not found very deep or extensive articulations of the idea of humanity and its dignity other than Kant's guiding one, but this is what we need. The UN Universal Declaration of Human Rights is one contemporary reference point. But being a political document and not a piece of moral philosophy, the Declaration vaults from the initial assertion of the inherent dignity of human beings to a sweeping manifesto of twenty-seven substantive rights. A contemporary proponent of human rights, the philosopher James Nickel, argues against theoretical compactness and in favor of a "many-legged" defense of human rights that interprets dignity as requiring all those "ways to recognize and respond to the value or worth that is found in life as a person," including "any particular feature of persons that has distinctive value" (Nickel 2005, 394). Nickel focuses on four sorts of moral claims secured by dignity: to have a life; to lead one's life; and to be free of severely cruel and degrading, as well as severely unjust, treatment. This goes in the right direction, although it does not give much guidance to those aspects of our humanity that comfort, move, and connect us but that are not so directly implicated in "leading" a life of one's own. Here the connection of dignity with full human agency remains strong.

Human capabilities theorists Amartya Sen and Martha Nussbaum introduce a more richly pluralistic picture of potentials for the full roster of characteristic human functionings. In Nussbaum's version, the one that most clearly articulates a particular vision of capabilities, the capabilities list has ten items ranging from life, bodily health, and integrity, through cognitive and emotional powers, to communion with nature, freedom to play, and a certain control over one's environment. This "thick" picture of human good is still very much oriented to agency through functionings, although it is decidedly more generous with respect to the range of functionings included. But "the list" remains a list, rather than an exploration of the diverse expressions and experiences of ourselves and others as human. Nussbaum simply annexes to this list bits of neo-Kantian machinery: that certain capabilities exert a "claim" that they should be realized and that each person exerts a claim as "an end" to the realization of her or his capabilities (Nussbaum 2000, 70-86, especially 74, 83). A more worrisome feature of this otherwise welcome pluralism about what is characteristically human is the disconcerting tendency of Nussbaum to refer to the absence of capabilities as the "absence of a human life," to describe one who lacks the capabilities for some functionings as "not really a human being" (73), or to characterize acts in the absence of certain capabilities as a "merely animal" way of life. But human beings are a complexly endowed kind of animal, and the idea of human dignity needs to capture and protect our humanity without erasing our animality. Nussbaum's more recent statements of her capabilities approach, in the 2006 book *Frontiers of Justice*, approach the relation between dignity and capabilities more carefully. Nussbaum now says that the capabilities themselves articulate the dignity of which a human being is *worthy*, and that a human life is inescapably that of an animal body with a developmental trajectory and persistent vulnerability. Even in the more recent work, however, Nussbaum persists in describing some severely incapacitated human lives as "not fully human" or "not a human life at all" conflating the normative role of the capabilities in prescribing acceptable treatment of human beings with a use of the capabilities list as a criterion to qualify or disqualify the humanity of some humans (Nussbaum 2006).

I am suggesting that we need space for an account that fully *naturalizes* the idea of the dignity of human beings, finding dignity not only in the rational agency of those human individuals who can be fully accountable (or in enough ways independently capable of functioning) but within a larger field of relations and responses. The relations and responses that are important are those that join us in what human beings recognize as particularly human modes of connection, what Eva Kittay describes as "a matrix of relationships embedded in social practices" in and through which we learn responses, responsibilities, and feelings that embody appropriate acknowledgments (Kittay 2005, 111). Dignity must refer to a standing in which human beings are free from, and actively shielded from, a variety of treatments, environments, and human relations incompatible with what dignity protects. Treatments incompatible with dignity include those that deny the presence of humanity in a human individual, such as relegating some human "kinds" to inferior grades of humanity or subhuman status, as has been so commonly done in human societies based on gender or racial or ethic categories (Walker 2003). They include ones that denigrate human beings for displaying attributes that are in fact inescapably human as if they are something "lower" than human (being vulnerable physically and psychologically or displaying need, fear, or pain) and ones that exploit a human attribute so as to denigrate a human individual (in the extreme case forms of torture, and more commonly exploitation through the needs of human beings). One case of exploiting a human attribute to denigrate a human being which we cannot take lightly, given its long history and social impact, is the common philosophical habit of declaring some particular characteristic human property as definitive or constitutive of humanity. By consequence of such stipulations, the humanity of a human individual who lacks that property or its fullest development may be denied, or the individual lacking the property may be declared not fully human, or of a lower grade of humanity, or (commonly) is simply ignored for the purposes of theoretical discussion (see Reader 2007; Kittay 2009). But dignity must also refer to the affirmation and positive and enabling support for the varieties of what is human, as well as openness to the enjoyment by and among human beings of what is human.

Capacities for rational choice, autonomous action, and moral responsibility are distinctive human attributes, and treating human beings who possess these valuable human attributes as if they did not, exploiting those attributes to denigrate human individuals, or aiming at the destruction and thwarting of those attributes does deny or assault human dignity. But the human characteristics that call upon the responsibility of accountable others are not exhausted by the rational capacity for accountability. Responsibility is called upon by human capacities for and vulnerabilities to many kinds of pain, suffering, insult, terror and neglect, as well as responsiveness of human beings to experiences of comfort, pleasure, physical integrity, skill, and control; by human capacities to respond to and to evoke and sustain shared or pleasurable or caring responses in others through touch, voice, feeling, shared attention, laughter or weeping; by the capacity to give and respond specifically to care, kindness, recognition, and fellow feeling (Kittay 2005, 122). Other characteristics that call out the responsibility of accountable agents are the humanly familiar kinds of expressiveness, absorption, and possessiveness that reveal human attachment, imagination, and memory, often in strikingly individual form. Human expressiveness includes but is not limited to capacities for more or less intentional self-representation. Much of what we love, enjoy, and are moved by in others, and what we long to feel is loved and cherished in ourselves and capable of moving others, are familiar and sometimes individuating features–physical, emotional, expressive–that have little to do with our rational capacities as agents but everything to do with our human purchase on others and our irreplaceability as human beings. (See also Vanlaere and Gastmans 2007).

### Relational dignity

Second, we need a fully *relational* way of conceiving and using the idea of dignity. Eva Kittay says that it is a mistake to sort individuals for moral consideration by intrinsic properties rather than by the relational property of being a member of the human family (Kittay 2005, 124). Annelies van Heijst argues that while the idea of intrinsic dignity should be retained, we need nonetheless to think of dignity as "secured, or even produced, in an interactive process of attentive caregiving" (van Heijst 2006a, 91). She quotes Paul Valadier saying that dignity in this sense "is a relationship, or rather, it manifests itself in the gesture by which we relate to others to consider them human, just as human as we are..." (94). I have already suggested that there are multiple characteristic features of human beings that are exercised and that are acknowledged in the kind of expression and recognition that constitutes dignity as an interpersonally effective standing. I want to say it is our humanity, in its varied expressions and enactments, that constitutes our claim to dignity, but that dignity is a *claim* that may or may not be honored. It is the affirmative response to the valid claim that constitutes the standing that is dignity. This is why it is comprehensible to speak of individuals' dignity being denied.

### Differentiating responses to dignity

Finally, when I speak of the need for a *differentiated* conception of dignity I refer not only to the varieties of human characteristics, expressions, and functions that we share and can acknowledge or affirm in other human beings, but to the varieties of response through which we can affirm or deny, celebrate or denigrate, support or thwart the humanity of these and their bearers. Dignity has been tightly linked to a particular kind of morally significant response: the attitude of respect that recognizes the moral personality and agency of others. It is not news that the attitude of respect, while it can be given a more extensive meaning, is heavily weighted toward non-interference in the exercise of rational self-control in those capable of it. The association between autonomy, negative liberty, noninterference, and dignity runs deep and runs in several directions through moral and political thought in the European and especially in the American tradition. But the idea that respect is the only or the primary attitude that constitutes the uptake of dignity is as exclusive as is the idea of dignity premised on rational agency to which it corresponds.

Assaults on dignity can take the forms of indifference, neglect, exclusion, ridicule, rejection, devaluation, and implicit as well as aggressive contempt. These are *failures* of human beings to meet others' humanity with forms of affirmation, confirming expression, communion, attention, and enjoyment. Annelies van Heijst comments at one point on disturbing reports from Dutch nursing homes, saying simply: "Practically no one spends some time with them, sits with them, talks to them or caresses them" (van Heijst 2006a, 90). It is remarkable how hard it remains theoretically to make the idea of human dignity responsive to such simple but urgent ways humanity can be denied, insulted, ignored and erased. There are nuanced physical and emotional responses that confirm a human presence–a greeting, a smile, a gaze, a touch. To meet with none of them or too few can be a profound offense to dignity. And it is a common feature of the intentional denial or instrumentalization of others' humanity–whether in concentration camps and prisons, or in nursing homes or other institutional environments–that efforts are made to render some distinctly human or especially humanly individuating aspects of a human presence obscure or deniable.

## 4. Conclusion: A twenty-first century agenda

We might hope that fundamental moral theory in the twenty-first century will move beyond pervasive fictions of equal rational actors in symmetrical relations and will tax itself with the problems of asymmetry in so many human relations. Asymmetrical relations of power and dependency require us to explain and defend the central moral value of keeping human beings in humanly dignifying relations to each other. One problem of asymmetry arises in the universal human situation of various forms of dependency, interdependency, and vulnerability; a second is the persistent fact of social subordination, inequality, or exclusion of, or spasms of persecution and violence toward, some groups of human beings by others. These problems place different demands, but I have suggested that at their root lies a strenuous task: to rethink the moral ideal of dignity that grounds demands for full recognition of the full humanity of every human individual and for truly humane responses to the humanity of others.

# 12.

# *Relationship based care and recognition Part one: sketching good care from the theory of presence and five entries*

Andries Baart and Frans Vosman

"Recognition" is the neglected moral pivot in discussions on the quality of care. In this article, the first of a series of two, we will explain and underpin this central idea by introducing a theoretical framework developed by Andries Baart, i.e. the theory of presence, and will clarify the choice of our perspective—a mixture of patient centeredness and systemic awareness. In the second article we will further elaborate on the question "what makes care good care" according to the theory of presence; this article is interrupted twice by interludes on the internal relation of good care and recognition. Thus we will contribute to the discussion on the quality of care, a search for quality that has become a search for technical provision. In this discussion the practical and fundamental moral aspects of quality of care have been obscured, to the detriment of the concept of quality of care itself.

## 1. The theory of presence

Professional social workers and health care workers stick to a characteristic way of handling social problems. Usually they try to reformulate stagnation in a client's life, opening it up for theory-driven diagnosis. In so doing, they change the client's acting—often chaotic and failing—into a rather orderly, well-defined problem that can be situated in a systematic, construed configuration of the understanding of causes, effects and remedies. As a rule, solutions are a compromise between what the client wishes to achieve and what can be done, controlled or reasonably predicted methodically. In order to induce the solution, the social worker brings some expertise to the client system, according to the previously determined plan, and only temporarily, in this way guaranteeing an efficient, effective and competent procedure. Having thus "intervened," he or she withdraws as soon as the job is done, or time and money are spent; in the worst case, the intervention may be unsuccessful and the case may appear hopeless.

Though more detailed distinctions and precision are possible, it will not be difficult to recognise in this picture the average care provider and social worker, and, more generally, the methodology of their care giving. This is approximately how the physician works, as does the welfare worker, health visitor, district nurse, youth helper, urban renovator, community organizer, community center worker, educator, rehabilitation officer, and so on. Even the pastor adopts this course of action. Most have been trained in this tradition and are paid to stick to this intervention approach. This approach enjoys a sufficient rate of success and therefore has significant social value.

Nevertheless, there is a very different way of handling social problems, or of meeting the need for care, called "the presence approach." In this article it will be presented as a preferable methodology, offering advantages that have been neglected of late. Its difference from the earlier-mentioned "intervention approach" is striking. The views and arguments as developed in the theory of presence rest heavily on empirical researches and case-studies (done by Baart and others, from the early nineties until now) carried out in several poor and disadvantaged neighborhoods and districts. The research was carried out in the fields of care for addicted and homeless adults and youngsters, multi-problem families and vulnerable, neglected or abused children, people suffering from HIV/AIDS in South Africa, frail residents in nursing homes and homes for the elderly, and migrant kids and their parents on children's playgrounds. In this empirical, and mostly longitudinal, research we are more interested in how care is provided and how good—or even excellent—care providers *apparently* proceed than in the analysis of social and behavioral problems of the care seekers. The focus is very much on what precisely is going on in the process of caring.

Although the presence approach has many different faces, styles and forms depending on the field where it is applied, there are some common, general traits. It is characteristic of "presence practitioners" that they *are there for* others without focusing directly on problem solving. Problem solving can indeed emerge from their efforts, but that is not their overt intention nor is problem solving the criterion of success. The most important thing these presence practitioners bring is the faithful offering of themselves: being there, making themselves available and providing the care that *turns out* to be needed. The underlying effort is to reach out and make the transition from "being there *with*" to "being there *for*," acknowledging that fruitful and relevant being there for someone includes an understanding from a "within perspective," that is a perspective taken within this particular relation.

In resource-poor neighbourhoods, presence practitioners are running errands, coming along to visit and listen, having a coffee or sharing a meal, completing a small household chore with someone, accompanying another to a doctor's appointment, going for a walk together. Countless examples could apply. Many of these forms of outreach are less rosy than one possibly assumes. At times the neighborhood presence practitioners are present to severe domestic violence, problems stemming from addiction, and structural problems that threaten communities as a whole. Probably there is little inclination to describe their rather informal conduct as "professional," let alone put it on a par with the social interventions mentioned earlier. But it is important to keep in mind that the presence approach does not orient itself towards solving identified problems as such. *Instead the focus is primarily on the cultivation of caring relationships, in which it may become clear what is morally desirable, what could be feasible, what may fit into that specific life and what the aspirations are.* This kind of understanding is also relevant to professional in such disciplines as medicine, nursing and education.

Furthermore it is characteristic that by design the presence approach operates as much as possible without a predetermined, narrowly defined professional identity, agenda or focus of attention. Preferably it gains form and content from open, multidimensional interactions[1], which over time grow into trusting relationships. In the context of maintaining and deepening such relationships, the presence practitioners normally come into contact with the integral social systems of the care receivers, such as their neighborhood, family and friends. Resources, including those needed to understand the life and aspirations of the care receiver, are found primarily within these meaningful social networks. In the course of this slowly developing association there emerges an articulation of hopes, pain, shortcomings, satisfactions and needs. Insofar as one can speak of the objectives of the presence approach, they come directly out of this process of gradual articulation. The actual design of the care provided, then, comes as the result of long-lasting, open-ended processes and not as the product of plans developed ahead of time. We know by now, from our further research, that these articulations which result from a relationship-based approach may occur instantly and don't necessarily need a *long* relationship. What seems to be crucial is the *aiming at* a relationship, as the presence approach does, even with the speechless, the demented, the mentally handicapped or the comatose patient. In good care the relationship is itself caring, beneficial and not purely instrumental.

Often the problems that the presence practitioners encounter are—regardless of whether we believe it or not—simply insoluble and some people turn out to be incorrigible. Some problems need nearly endless amounts of time. Other problems relate to the tragedy and the contingency that are part of life itself. Their solutions cannot be hastened as they concern "slow questions" (existential issues) to which no quick answers can be manufactured (Kunneman 2005). Other problems again are so firmly embedded that they seem likely to pass only with the generation itself. For such problems, the monomaniacal determination to eliminate problems hastily (through the power of subsidies, programs, new techniques) has the potential to be counterproductive and even destructive. As Annelies van Heijst states in several publications: they tend to add to suffering (instead of relief). In that context, a trusted and familiar figure who knows how to listen attentively is worth more than an expert prattler, professional newspeak or the continuous reinventing of intervention programs whose history seems to be lost in the mists of time. Without giving in to passivity and defeatism, it must be acknowledged that some problems offer no hope of resolution, and it can be of great help to be able to acknowledge as much without the professional needing to withdraw, or without recourse to "skimming"—restricting professional care to those who have the best chance of improving.

Although in hospital nursing, in the care for the elderly in nursing homes or for drug dependent visitors in shelters the characteristics of presence care differ—slightly or more profoundly—their main feature is still the same: *the care provided arises from relationship based programming*. The following catchwords belong to its overall methodology: patience, attentiveness and receptivity; relational matching, virtue and competence driven dedication ("don't leave them alone") and the ability to give attention to most severe problems in the little everyday things of life ("diluted seriousness"). The presence practitioner makes free but professional use of rather loose and mixed forms of contact that attach themselves closely to the ordinary patterns of daily life, adhering to rhythms, social structures and the prevailing language of the care seekers.

The presence approach is not a wonder drug and renders superfluous very little of the existing apparatus of social intervention help provision. Presence practitioners have time and take time, and they work to ensure that the time available remains "free" (i.e., not filled in advance with professional plans and targets). From this standpoint they get to know people and their environment more deeply and find themselves better prepared to assess what is at hand. They are also in a strong position to share history and build trust with care seekers. They know and are known by the people they work for and thus are able to understand, on multiple levels, their personal history and the local dynamics and are able to contribute to those dynamics in a rich way.

Contained within the values and philosophy of the presence approach is a sharp critique of the bureaucratic violence that "the poor" (the frail, vulnerable, unwanted ones) undergo, whereby their story, their dignity and their "problem" (the only things they possess that bestow an identity on them) are all too often too quickly and easily dispensed with. Bureaucrats, apparently, know better, and too often they are lousy listeners. However reasonable, fair and efficient a bureaucracy strives to be, the weakest members of society rarely experience it that way. In the theory of presence, bureaucracy as such isn't criticized but (the pitfall of, or at least tendency to) the *self referential character of modern care systems* that imposes its logic, interests, and rhythm upon the care receiver as a more or less subtle institutional pressure, or as social-technological interventionism rooted in a very one-sided rationality and restricted morality. The theory of presence is firmly based upon the ethics of care and in that frame a dozen minor theories are applied to the theory of presence itself: theories on processes of matching, on consolation and loneliness, on engagement and social inclusion, on propinquity and (professionally) being like a friend, on reflective professionalism and rule driven behaviour, on the active and leaving mode of professional proceedings, on powerlessness to fate and tragedy, on open attentiveness, on kinds of legitimacy of interventions, on different types of estrangement and distancing oneself, on the value of evidence-based and practice-based or wisdom-based knowledge and so on. The presence theory starts where descriptions and analyses of practice end, and tries in social-scientific, philosophical and theological terms to specify why and in what respect the presence approach works and is of value, and which understanding of common humanity it implies.

In short, the presence theory encompasses a professional way of doing (methodology), a cultural critique, an explicit normative perspective on care, a paradigmatic shift in producing relevant and sound knowledge about care giving, and a characteristic interpretation of societal injustice and human suffering (and human dignity). Certainly, the presence theory is much more than a new alternative method. It may be interpreted as the (nowadays frequently forgotten and pushed aside) basis of all interventionistic intention—its critical memory, its ultimate legitimacy and its proper frame of relevance (that is, what it is all about).

Since its publication in the Netherlands in 2001, the theory of presence has had a warm, if sometimes critical, welcome (putting into words what so many people already felt but couldn't articulate nor provide alternative explanations of) and has gradually grown into a success, both in practice and in theory. It became more and more elaborate, e.g. evolving an institutional and managerial perspective. And its relevance was tested in domains of care and welfare where "being present" seemed at face value to be very difficult or even impossible. Nowadays several longitudinal field experiments in various domains of care are carried out and closely researched. Prominent scholars and many students (MA and PhD) have contributed to the development of the theory.

## 2. Sketching good care: from which point of view?

In the next paragraph we will be looking for an answer to the question: what makes normal, common care good care? So, criteria for the *quality of care* are at stake. The question is an urgent and relevant one with an explicit political and normative point, and it goes beyond detached scientific analysis. Criteria for the quality of good care may be arrived at from very different point of views. Before presenting the perspective of the presence approach we will consider five (types of) "entries" to the debate.

### *Entry 1: Objective needs*

In the case of the South African HIV/AIDS pandemic and the associated sense of emergency, good care tends to be restricted to fundamental (or basic) means and needs. It is all about good medication, safe sex and healthy food. But what do we mean by "fundamental" or "basic"? Is antiretroviral medicine more fundamental than bread, than grants for children, decent funerals, or education for vulnerable children and women? Is it more basic and necessary than personal, attentive proximity, and treatment with honour or respect? Obviously there is a bottom line: without life, all talk about rights, education and respectfulness is pointless, but as soon as we rise above that absolute bottom line we are in trouble.

One may, of course, try to return to the "objective" determination of human needs, but the best-known attempts to do so (see Maslow 1999 and his successors), have been heavily criticized for their cultural bias and failure to account for people who, in many respects, turn out to be the most interesting subjects—that is, those outstanding in morals, sports, arts and craftsmanship. A simple example may illustrate the defectiveness of this kind of reasoning differently: if the poor need bread, why should we not shove it in their face? After all, objectively they get what they want. But clearly the poor need more than bread: they need bread *given in a specific way*, with respect and without denigration. Being hungry can be preferable to the loss of self-respect. This conclusion is essential in the process of understanding what makes care good care.

We would argue that there is no uncontradicted, social-scientific theory or generally accepted ethical theory by which we may escape the moral and political discussions of the criteria of good care. It is rather an objective of an ethical theory to absorb those discussions.

### *Entry 2: Foundation standards*

Another way to discover what obviously counts as good care, finds one looking at the education of healthcare professionals: Here one may observe how they are instructed in their vocational training, what is said to matter, what a professional healthcare worker should do, know and be according to the standards of good care. Here we find the actual standards of care as they are transferred to novices. When standards of good care are equated to the accountability criteria of the *foundation standards* that healthcare professionals should meet, the next picture is clear[2]. Healthcare professionals will

1. ... know the academic subject matter required for proficiency within their area. They will use this knowledge as needed in their role.

2. … know the various methods of giving and obtaining information. They will communicate effectively, both orally and in writing.
3. … will understand how their role fits into their department, their organization and the overall healthcare environment. They will identify how key systems affect services they perform and quality of care.
4. … understand how employability skills enhance their employment opportunities and job satisfaction. They will demonstrate key employability skills and will maintain and upgrade skills, as needed.
5. ... understand the legal responsibilities, limitations, and implications of their actions within the healthcare delivery setting. They will perform their duties according to regulations, policies, laws and legislated rights of clients.
6. ... understand accepted ethical practices with respect to cultural, social, and ethnic differences within the healthcare environment. They will perform quality healthcare delivery.
7. ... understand the existing and potential hazards to clients, co-workers, and self. They will prevent injury or illness through safe work practices and follow health and safety policies and procedures.
8. ... understand the roles and responsibilities of individual members as part of the healthcare team, including their ability to promote the delivery of quality healthcare. They will interact effectively and sensitively with all members of the healthcare team.
9. ... understand the fundamentals of wellness and the prevention of disease processes. They will practice preventive health behaviors among the clients.
10. ... apply technical skills required for all career specialties. They will demonstrate skills and knowledge as appropriate.
11. ... use information technology applications required within all career specialties. They will demonstrate use as appropriate to healthcare applications.

Good care according to these standards (and similar ones in the domains of nursing, youth health care, social work etc.) is totally disconnected from what the care receiver might ask, experience or want to reject; Good care is specified in the formal terms of adequate professional interventions *related to the thing, the problem, the disease.* In a way which is different from the first entry, this entry also aims at "objective" criteria, not derived from universal human needs, but from universal standards of good problem solving.

### *Entry 3: Consumers' experiences*

In the Netherlands good care (for the elderly, and in many respects also for children, mentally handicapped people, psychiatric patients and so on) is defined in the so called *Quality Assurance Framework for Accountable Care* (*Kwaliteitskader Verantwoorde Zorg*[3]) and in several white papers elaborating that framework in specific aspects. The *Quality Assurance Framework for Accountable Care* has been developed by ActiZ[4] together with other stakeholders. It is a standard that measures the quality of care and also ensures transparency. It objectively and structurally maps care performance and the quality of care that clients experience. A Dutch website is available where visitors can check the quality of care that individual companies provide and the distinctive features of that care.

"Accountable care" and the processes and performances that produce accountable care are rooted in the ideal (or assumption or assignment) of the care receiver's free choice and self regulation, both simple translations of "autonomy." In order to facilitate these, communication and information on relevant subject matters are provided to the patient; in addition, preferences of or agreements with the patient on his or her treatment and lifestyle are recorded in a personal care plan. This has become a *conditio sine qua non.* No care without a personal care plan. Those plans cover four domains of care:

- physical wellbeing (bodily care, health promotion, protection, good food etc.),
- comfortable living conditions (adequate housing, feeling "at home," safe environment),

- participation (being invited into meaningful activities—instead of being passive and without a say), and finally
- mental wellbeing (having the opportunity to be on your own, being prevented from psychiatric illness (depression) and being able to live according to one's (religious) values).

Each of these four domains of accountable care is made operational and "measurable" in dozens of specifications that are closely linked to tightly defined professional interventions and organizational conditions. Thus a comprehensive care quality system is designed out of a *formal* but *encompassing* philosophy of *accountable* care. Its claim is that all aspects of neediness are covered, and in that sense it is a total system.

It provides the care system with a formal set of focus points that can, and even must, be used to constantly improve care. The principal way of doing so, is the (bi)annual measurement of care quality by the so called CQ-index (Customer Quality Index). Those surveys are derived from the CAHPS surveys[5], which are similar to patient satisfaction surveys but are not the same. CQ-surveys include ratings of providers and health plans but go beyond this type of question by asking patients and consumers to report on their experiences with health care services *as conceptualized in the above mentioned four domains*. In order to support valid comparisons and benchmarking across the Dutch national health care system, the surveys are standardized as it comes to (a) the instruments (same questions), (b) the protocol (same way of collecting data), (c) the analysis (same way of interpreting the findings) and (d) the reporting. The comparability makes the information useful for quality improvement as well as public reporting. Reporting is done in a National Benchmarking Database[6]: here consumers may inform themselves before choosing a hospital, treatment or residence. As a matter of fact, it is here that subsidizing agencies find the legitimation for stopping or continuing their finance. The benchmark is comparative, not objective: the quality of care in a specific setting is good, average or bad *compared to other care providers*, not to an objective quality standard (although it is the intention to find or construe one). Three major programs are executed in conjunction with the benchmark[7]: improvement, development and innovation of care. Those (huge) national programs provide many professional training facilities, databases of best practices, grants for innovation, professional workshops, "knowledge networks" and so on. And, finally, once again those care quality improvement programs are monitored and investigated by impressive, academic research programs.

This quality system heavily dominates the care-providing institutions in the Netherlands; it leaves hardly any room for alternative approaches and more substantial views on care. From our point of view, specific characteristics of this quality system should be criticized. These are the underlying idea of autonomy of the patient (what about the obvious vulnerability of that very same patient?), the formal and non-substantial standards of care quality (with no or little room for the beneficence of being seen, honoured, respected, relationally included), the absence of moral reasoning and the prevailing improvement of the technical aspects of care giving that are social. We would also include the attendant risk of window dressing (having a main focus on good benchmark scores instead of good care itself[8]) and the one-sided emphasis on quantitative measurements at the expense of patients' narratives and also of professional narratives.

### *Entry 4: Radically patient centred*

"The standard definition of quality now recognised internationally is that of the US Institute of Medicine which has six criteria: patient-centered, safe, effective, timely, efficient, and equitable (Institute of Medicine 2001[9]). Today, *patient-centered* seems to have become the term of choice in the quality improvement literature (occasionally supplanted by 'patient and family-centered care') despite the fact that there are problems associated with it." This quotation from *Seeing the person in the patient*[10] (Goodrich and Cornwell 2008, 19/20) symbolizes a turning point in the quality of care debate: good care is, to start with, patient-centered. The Institute of Medicine's definition of patient centered care incorporates both the "what" of process and the "how" of relationship, attitudes and behaviors. The definition has six dimensions:

1. Compassion, empathy and responsiveness to needs, values and expressed preferences

2. Co-ordination and integration

3. Information, communication and education

4. Physical comfort

5. Emotional support, relieving fear and anxiety

6. Involvement of family and friends.

Although we may notice similarities to the "domains of care" mentioned above, the *differences* are more striking, not least because of dimensions one and six. The UK report (24/25, 29) not only specifies the theoretical meaning of being patient centered but also investigates what different people say about it. Typically, politicians paint broad and ambitious visions of patients' experience of care and then translate the visions into practical pledges or targets that focus on a *limited sub-set* of the six dimensions of patient-centered care. Managers, educationalists, professional leaders and officers of patient organisations define patient-centered (very) *differently*. Hospital staff prefer *ordinary, human words* when referring to (good) care, for example, respect, dignity, sensitive, understanding, gentle, kind, welcome, friendly, comfort, smile, compassion and communication. "Seeing the person in the patient" resonates positively with staff and managers at all levels. Expressions aiming at the same standards of quality can be found in the works of Annelies van Heijst, Mieke Grypdonck and Andries Baart.

The more radical and more detailed elaboration of this kind of criteria of quality of care, can be found in literature on "nursing and presence." In a review article, written by Holly Covington, the following table is presented (Covington 2005, 170) summarizing explicit or implicit examples of caring presence in literature, where presence is depicted as the eminent form of good care (Table 1).

| Author(s) | Perspective |
|---|---|
| Paterson and Zderad | Reciprocal relationship of availability, openness, mutuality and intimacy |
| Watson | Conscious awareness in the relationship, resulting in connection between patient and nurse |
| Roach | Quality of compassion that allows sharing |
| Pettigrew | Availability and self-giving, listening with tangible awareness, and becoming willingly involved with another who is suffering |
| Horner | Requires full awareness, receptivity, and attention to the other |
| Ray | Way of engaging and interacting within the process of caring inquiry |
| Swanson-Kauffman | A way to share in meanings, feelings, and experiences of the one being cared for |
| Gilje | Attending to another in an intersubjective and intrasubjective exchange of energy that transforms into a meaningful experience |
| Hines | Being available as a unique human being in which there is an exchange of authentic, meaningful awareness; essence linking; and ultimate realization of human potential |
| Parse | Being with and attentive to the person during the process of becoming |
| Euswas | Being there and mindfully present results in intersubjective connectedness |
| Boykin and Schoenhofer | Way of being within a caring-healing relationship that allows interconnectedness, making it possible to learn, grow, and transcend suffering |
| Osterman and Schwartz-Barcott | Four ways of being there, with focused energy that reflects varying degrees of intensity |

| Author(s) | Perspective |
|---|---|
| Doona et al | Intersubjective existential experience in which the nurse encounters the patient as a unique human being in a unique situation and chooses to "spend" self on behalf of patient |
| Godkin | A 3-stage process within the nurse-patient interaction; may result in greater patient satisfaction |
| Covington | A way of being and relating |

Table 1: Explicit or implicit examples of caring presence.

We point out the shift from "patient centered" to "relational": it is a subtle but essential change. The meta-synthesis of presence in nursing literature by Deborah Fingeld-Connett (2006), results in the following figure (711); Figure 1.

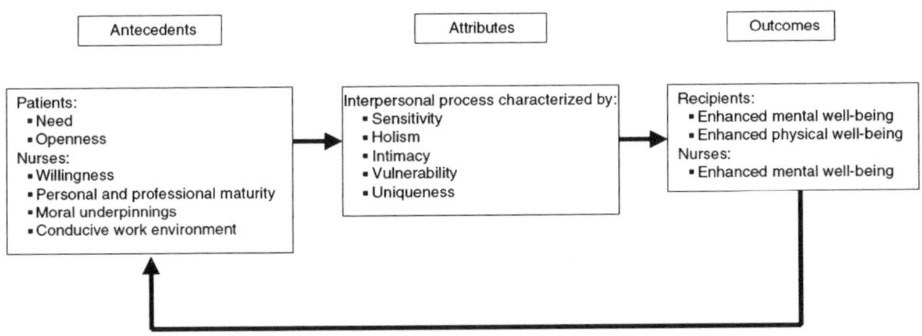


Figure 1: Meta-synthesis of presence in nursing literature.

Here, the penury of the patient, the professional and personal characteristics of the caregiver and interpersonal process variables contribute jointly to the outcome of good care, both in the experience of the recipients and the caregivers. Of course this type of care quality criteria is rather "soft," compared to the rigorous CQ-system, but it is morally and substantially more "loaded": it looks for care quality related to the quality of the caring *relation*. Although not yet proved to be so, it may be more effective and cheaper.

## *Entry 5: From good care to politics*

Before presenting our views and hypotheses, we should point out that this is neither the first nor the only attempt to articulate criteria for good care inductively. In Baart's *Een theorie van de presentie* (2001 /2004[3], 650-664, paragraph 1.2.1) he made a phenomenological reconstruction of the (ingredients of the) request for help. What do people ask for when they ask for help? It was discovered that that question consists of nine specific and ordered elements, which are analyzed step-by-step and in detail. Those elements are:

(1) Does it matter, (2) to you, (3) that this, (4) here (5) to me (6) always (7) happens in this way, (8) hurts and (9) should end? The first thing is: Does it matter? (and not: Please, free me!) That is a request for recognition. And further: Does it matter—not in general, not for an abstract institution, but for a human being I can see, feel and address? Does "*it*" matter, not as an abstract issue, or a well and bureaucratically categorized illness, defect or right that is out of control and beyond understanding (chaotic, mighty, repetitive), but as, rather, something concrete and tangible, regardless of what it is called or how it is classified. And then, the final elements: It hurts and it should stop; please, help me. This phenomenologically reconstructed question is subsequently analyzed in respect of its tensions, professional viability, etc. The last step of the analysis is the most relevant one in this context. Each of these elements matches a specific political claim, or to put it another way, with normative criteria for good, just and "careful" politics / government. Here we find the "translation" of the ideal-typical request for help into political criteria of good care. In Table 2 the question and criteria are summarized.

| **Elements of the request for help** | **Good social politics gives, respects or safeguards the care receiver's...** |
|---|---|
| Does it matter | Right(s) |
| To you | Normative-reflective professionals |
| That this | Identity (singularity) |

| Elements of the request for help | Good social politics gives, respects or safeguards the care receiver's... |
|---|---|
| Here | Situatedness (framework) |
| To me | Political power and say |
| Always | Lived coherence of life |
| Happens in this way | Means, facilities and knowledge |
| Hurts | Voice and language |
| And should end? | Time, rhythm and meaning |

Table 2: The answer to the question for help (freely after Table 45.124.2 in TP, 662-663).

This article may also be interpreted as the attempt to rearticulate operationally these findings and conclusions (including Baart 2003b).

## Notes

[1] After the completion of A *theory of presence* Baart wrote several supplementary studies, e.g. on open attentiveness, trust, vulnerability etc. See the references at the end of this volume.

[2] These criteria are quoted from http://www.nde.state.ne.us/healthscience/nationalhsstandards.htm (Nebraska Department of Education; visited Feb, 21st 2009).

[3] This report has been developed gradually, from 'On our way to norms for accountable care' (2005) and 'Norms for accountable care' (2006) to 'Quality assurance framework for accountable care' (2007); see: http://www.zorgvoorbeter.nl/kwaliteitskader/verpleging-verzorging-en-zorg-thuis-vvt/ and http://www.zorgvoorbeter.nl/kwaliteitskader/verpleging-verzorging-en-zorg-thuis-vvt/visie-en-achtergrond/normen-verantwoorde-zorg1/. The policy is described on: http://www.actiz.nl/opinies-en-beleid/kwaliteit/30/148 (visited Feb. 21st 2009).

[4] ActiZ is the Dutch trade association and employers' organization for providers of care and other services - at home, at residential homes for the elderly or at homes for the elderly and nursing homes, and at infant and child health clinics; see: http://www.actiz.nl/actueel/branchenieuws/42/67 (visited Feb. 21st 2009).

[5] Consumer Assessment of Healthcare Providers and Systems, see: https://www.cahps.ahrq.gov/default.asp and see (in Dutch) http://www.zonmw.nl/nl/onderwerpen/alle-programma-s/meten-patientenervaringen (visited Feb. 20th 2009).

[6] See: http://www.kiesbeter.nl (visited Feb. 20th 2009).

[7] See: http://www.zorgvoorbeter.nl and http://www.zonmw.nl/nl/onderwerpen/alle-programma-s/zorg-voor-beter/ (visited Feb. 20th 2009).

[8] This critique has been spelled out by CEG (Centre for Ethics and Health / Centrum voor ethiek en gezondheid) in the white paper *Passend bewijs. Ethische vragen bij het gebruik van evidence in het zorgbeleid* (2008), see: http://www.ceg.nl/cgi-bin/publ.pl?id=433&type=4 (visited Feb. 21st 2009).

[9] See: http://www.iom.edu/CMS/8089/5441.aspx (visited Feb. 21st 2009).

[10] Free download: http://www.kingsfund.org.uk/publications/the_kings_fund_publications/the_point_of_care.html

# 13.

# *Relationship based care and recognition Part two: good care and recognition*

Frans Vosman and Andries Baart

"Recognition" is the neglected moral pivot in discussions on the quality of care. In this article, the second of a series of two, we will elaborate on the question "what makes care good care" according to the theory of presence as developed by Andries Baart. This article is interrupted twice by interludes on the internal relation of good care and recognition. In this way we will contribute to the discussion on the quality of care, a search for quality that has become a search for technical provision. In this discussion practical and fundamental moral aspects of the quality of care have been obscured, to the detriment of the concept of the quality of care itself.

This article builds on the first in the series where we introduced the theory of presence, and clarified the choice of our perspective, that of a mixture of patient centeredness and systemic awareness.

## What makes care good care?

What makes care good care?[1] We would answer:

1. It must have a proper identity: it must actually *be* care.
2. It must be relevant: fine-tuned to specified needs.
3. It must be true, that is, effective.
4. It must be legitimate in more respects than just the legal.
5. It must be do-able, technically and humanly speaking.
6. Good care is beneficence, a caring good in itself and *sui generis*.

These six criteria will be elucidated and analyzed in the next six paragraphs.

## 1. Care that deserves to be called care

To understand what care is, we prefer not to start from ethical or philosophical literature[2] but from the colloquial language. "Care" in Dutch has, in certain respects, the same meaning as in English, but there are significant differences, as is the case with the German "Sorge" (Fürsorge, besorgen). Regardless of the formal meaning, there is in the Netherlands today a trendy use of the term "care." Even the car dealership gives one (with regard to his car) a "passport to care" and the housemaid is called an "interior care-taker." The whole social domain of "social work," in fact, is referred to as the "sector of care and welfare," which includes therapy, hospitals, education, geriatric help, community organizing, child protection, etc.: a motley collection. But we know that there are caregivers outside this domain and there are professionals within the domain who obviously are—compared to our quality standards of care—*not* care-givers, but simply nurses and doctors doing their job. Stipulating what we mean by care is not a superfluous gesture (see Table 3).

| Aspects of care | Carrying out by | Typical quotation | The problem | The supplement to the situation | Intention |
|---|---|---|---|---|---|
| ***Caring (about)*** | 1 Minding | I care (I mind) what is happening. It matters to me. | Not being noticed (potential indifference) | Observation and commitment | Relating to (the other, the need) |
| | 2 (Anxious) concern or solicitude | I care (am concerned) about you | Accepted as moral appeal (thoughtless-ness) | Mercy / compassion | Being sensitive to the fate of the other |
| ***Care*** | 3 Readiness | Do you care (are you ready) to do such and such? | Uncertainty about the willingness to act | Motivation or drive to do anything | Developing the desire, the want, the inclination |

| Aspects of care | Carrying out by | Typical quotation | The problem | The supplement to the situation | Intention |
|---|---|---|---|---|---|
| *(Taking) care (of)* | 4 Attention | What is happening needs my constant care (attention) | Being at risk | Watch / guard | Noticing danger and if necessary: acting |
| | 5 Maintenance | I am caring for (maintaining) it so it will last | Continuity | Preservation | Keeping it in a good shape |
| | 6 Aid | With my care (aid) it can be accomplished | Deficiency | Repair / supplement | Problem solving; being of service |
| *(Providing) care for* | 7 (Professional) intervention | I am caring for (attending to / intervening on behalf of ) the wounded | Moral involvement (responsibility) | Competent help | Doing what is desirable |
| *(With) care* | 8 Caution | I will do it with care (carefully, cautiously) | Fragility | Tenderness & interest | Treasuring or at least avoiding harm |

Table 3: The meaning of "care."

These meanings are not mutually exclusive. On the contrary, they significantly overlap, defining, based on practical experience, not care as such, but *aspects* of care. Together they suggest the following:

- Care is the effort to keep life (existence) going when it is failing, weak, in pain, in danger, broken, threatened, fragile, and when it loses its quality, autonomy and self-sufficiency. Care and the (potential or factual) *discontinuity* of life are two sides of the same coin. Discontinuity here means: If life is left to itself and the forces constituent of its actual state, it will turn into something bad, undesirable, painful.

- Care is a *common, every day* activity with a very broad range of caring actions (not exclusively restricted to specialists, women, adults), not limited to specific "domains" (such as health), but applicable to every aspect of life; care is not even confined to life but applies to existence (including "things" such as vases, cars, wine and even dead people).
- Care is given before, during and after the endangerment of the continuity and is, consequently, *more than repairing* or putting things right after they have been disturbed.
- Care is a common, every day *activity*. This characteristic is rather problematic. No one can justly assert they care if they have nothing more than caring feelings and intentions ("I care about the poor: I am concerned about their situation but don't care to give money or take action"). In such cases we would say the caring is not genuine because it does not translate into action: No care is provided. Although care implies a specific state of mind, intention, readiness and concern, it is not that state of mind or moral inclination by itself. An "adequate" transition into action does not necessarily imply that good care has "good results"; the results of the action determine to a large extent whether my care has been adequate. A father who has done his utmost in caring for his infant child may yet confront the tragedy of crib death. Evidently, the care given has not been adequate, but is this person to blame? It depends on how adequately the care *could* have been taken—on what the care-giver could have and should have known. Compare this case to another: I take care of my terminally-ill father; he has some good days but nevertheless dies soon. The result of my care should not be situated in the yes / no (sooner or later) dying of my father, but in my contribution to the quality of life he experienced and the quality of his process of dying. In order to correctly evaluate the adequacy of the translation of concern into the care activity, one must relate the intention of the care (what good is aimed at?), the competence of execution and the experience of its results.

- All care is provided with reference to a desired state of life or to a preferred quality of existence: care is directed to bring about "good life." There is no absolute criterion: What may be valued as "good" or "good care" depends on the local appreciation of the threatened life / existence and on the locally valued qualities of that life. Care is a good to be discerned within relationships. This lack of an absolute criterion, of course, does not exclude the possible existence of absolute good, the good of human life and a good highly ranked in the hierarchy of goods, the good of a life of honour. Care needs *local validation* to know for sure that it is "care" and nothing else (such as meddlesomeness or self-centered interventions on the part of the so-called caregiver). "Local" is in this case highly correlated to the care receiver ('s experience / feedback). In this light, "good life" has more to do with "sensible life" than with "comfortable and undisturbed life." (Even a precious vase that is going to fall to pieces needs no care, *if*, for instance, those fragments are meant to be beautifully arranged in a museum and make sense again in their new identity.)
- Care needs the effort of an other and, taking our lead from Table 3, we may presume some of the crucial *characteristics of the care-giver*: they should relate to the problem (appeal), be sensitive, look closely at the problem in its specificity, become finely attuned to it; they should accept their role and responsibility, do the work competently and cautiously, be receptive to feedback (does it achieve the intended aim?). Care is clearly more than a technical problem-solving activity: it is moral, expressive (affectionate), social etc.
- Care needs, as we have said, the effort of *an other* and consequently touches upon the dependence of the care-receiver: their self-sufficiency falls short and they are "in need" of the help of another person. As caring is a common practice, this need of an other is also common; here the modern and hyperbolized interpretation of autonomy is criticised. The normal situation for social beings is not "autonomy" but mutual dependency and—

with Ricoeur—vulnerability. At the same time, it is important to point out that caring may induce (unhealthy) dependency and increase vulnerability.

With this short exploration we hope, beyond finding common ground, to come to a more fully developed, open and broad conceptualization of care than one usually finds. That broadness is already employed in common language and practice, but too often it is forgotten as soon as scientists and politicians come in.

Our first answer to the question "what makes care good care?" is: It should be care in a rich and profound sense. It should be care and nothing else, such as simple problem solving.

1. As follows from the exploration above, the criteria of good care can be boiled down to the experiences of the care receiver: good care is care *experienced* as good care—immediately or in the long run. If for instance care providers argue strongly and even convincingly that they have provided good care (timely, competent, safe, accessible, transparent etc.) but the care receiver feels neglected, humiliated, object of professional violence, treated as a number (regrettably all not imaginary!), we can hardly stick to the claim this was indeed good care. I would argue that the experiences of the care receiver have priority, without stating that this priority is absolute. The assessments or evaluations of the care receivers are not sacrosanct but should be investigated critically—nevertheless they embody the first criterion of good care.
2. This criterion of good care is rooted in the philosophy of the care receiver as a person (not as a locus of disease, deficiency, etc.) and by consequence as a co-creator of care provided—although frail, dependent, sometimes afraid and even dying. Care is not a product, created and delivered by one party and consumed by the other, but a mutual effort. Good care is aiming at that mutuality; values such as the human dignity and one's biographical situatedness (being someone in a unique way) are intrinsically interwoven in this intention.

In light of these reflections, let us now consider further what makes care good care: the other criteria are in many respects the elaboration of this first one.

## 2. Tuning

There is no good care, unless it is attuned to the need, the endangered quality, the continuity of life. Preferably, the care will be "well tuned," "fine tuned" or "adequately linked." But let us begin by focusing on tuning as such: What is involved in the tuning of care? We discern four dimensions.

### *A. Pragmatic*

Within the pragmatic dimension of tuning we concentrate on avoiding mismatches: which is to say, on overcoming the non-correspondence of (care) supply and (care) demand and failures to connect care and need correctly. From detailed, earlier analyses (Baart 2002a) we know that the failure to (at)tune is too often one-sidedly accounted for in terms of lacking facilities (no money, no priority, budget cuts and downsizing, elimination of services and expertise, etc.).

But besides this evident failure of tuning, there are more subtle problems: namely, deficient methods. In the present day, the provision of care is highly "methodized." Although the purpose of using methods based on the positive sciences and "evidence-based findings" (Van der Laan 2003; Melief 2003) is to improve the quality of care, such methods often bring restrictions that hinder fine-tuning. The unavoidable standardization—in combination with the severe control and monitoring of practitioners in order to force them to stick to the rules, protocols and other regulations inherent in the method used —interferes with the taking into account of specific characteristics of the situation, client and professional. Good care is conceptualized as the obedient application of general insights to the specific case, ruling out the freedom of the care giver to act according to their own understanding or "local learning processes." This well-ordered and thoroughly planned standardization has difficulty coming to terms with the chaotic life style so common among marginalized care seekers.

The third kind of mismatch goes deeper and does not concern facilities or methods but cultural obstacles to fine-tuning. Concisely formulated, in the provision of care we mostly see two different worlds come together: The world of the professional with its own rationality, bureaucratic logic, meticulous time management, and language, clashes with the life world of the care receiver, with the latter having to adjust on threat of receiving no care at all. The longer one works with "poor, vulnerable and marginalized people," the more one is convinced that this "cultural mismatch"—the almost unbridgeable gap between different ways of organizing life—is the most persistent and difficult mismatch to overcome. Care receivers—no matter how much they should be treated as fellow citizens—do not nearly so often meet the standards of the rational, deliberately choosing and deciding (Green and Shapiro 1994), orderly living patients they are supposed to be. Frequently they refuse to open their mail, don't arrive on time for appointments, or eat fatty and salty food; they spend money on things they would be better to avoid, drink alcohol when they shouldn't; often they choose the wrong husband or wife and don't bother to change their sedentary, passive lifestyle. This rarely matches the bureaucratic and professional logic that regulates their care.

Closely related to this is a fourth mismatch, which concerns the preponderance of conceptual power or knowledge-influence. The one who asks for care and help is in principle mistrusted and must prove that their request is justified and appropriate (that they are not cheating), whereas the doctor, the nurse, the researcher has undoubted insight and knowledge. Nine times out of ten the professional care giver's interpretation of what is going on is conceded as being more credible. The professional's account is assumed to be more plausible and well-informed. When push comes to shove, it is the professionals who win, and the sick, the poor, the addicted, the mad and the imprisoned are considered wrong. The same applies to the "street level bureaucracy." Those care givers, functioning right inside the world of the afflicted and employing the "feminine way of caring" (by far the greatest part of all care is provided by women), normally lose out to more highly placed (male) colleagues, such as the manager or the principal, who are less directly involved. Their "knowledge" is easily lost when presented one step up the hierarchy.

### *B. Phenomenological*

Tuning care to needs is more than successful pragmatic "calibration"; it has three other dimensions, beginning with a phenomenological one. Needs must be "disclosed" (Eikeland 2008, 128; 240). They must have the opportunity to show themselves—be it step-by-step, over the longer term, in an upside-down or back-to-front way, through dozens of tests, stories, lies, or otherwise. Professional carers think too easily that they understand what is needed or sought. But a closer look reveals that people seldom formulate their aspirations directly (Letiche 2008, 12). They feel ashamed or stupid, are not ready to trust the potential carer, or else want to save face (maintain their dignity or honour). They presume that certain questions will yield better outcomes, and may not even know their own desires, needing a longer-lasting and more trusting relationship to be clear about what they want and need. That's why we say tuning should include the process by which care receivers may find their voice, show their face, have the floor, occupy their rightful place in the public domain ("be someone"). Although giving care is an activity, it implies a disciplined passivity, a mode of letting (come), of waiting for what eventually will turn out (or not). Impatience and good care are mostly irreconcilable. Impatience often leads to the care giver doing what fulfils his or her own needs (such as taking away uneasy feelings). Even in so-called emergency cases some "passivity" is a prerequisite for good, well-tuned care.

### *Interlude 1: Recognition*

In the last decades care providing has shifted from "what we have to offer" to "what the consumer asks for," from "you have to take what we produce" to "we deliver what you want." Nevertheless in many cases care receivers don't ask questions: they dare not, they cannot, they suffer from shame, depleted self-confidence or they may be too sick, mentally handicapped or psychotic. They don't succeed in being critical consumers in the care market. Therefore, a *good* care provider should not only hear what is explicitly asked for but should also be sensitive to implicit appeals, aspirations and suffering and respond with care to what is not apparent in the care seeker's situation. The care giver, phenomenologically speaking, creates the space where these appeals may appear, come forward and show themselves. In so doing, a basic act of recognition—prior to all help and care—is accomplished:

- the suffering of the care-seeker is represented as *real* and the appeal is accepted: the care-seeker is not left alone (with feelings deemed to be not worth looking at);
- by this recognition, we see the rehabilitation of the care-seeker (he is not a fool, not unworthy and longing for help) and mutuality is installed: from now on, the suffering concerns both parties;
- what takes place is relational inclusion: recognition shows itself as a quality of the relationship;
- and from that moment on, the act of recognition has produced a shared reference: it has determined what that relationship is all about.

So the primary tasks of the recognizing party are:

- creating room for the care seeker so they can make themself known: inviting them to come into existence;
- unfolding the position obviously occupied and the identity obviously aimed at (the care-seeker asks to be recognized as teenage mother, caring husband, honest drug addict etc. and not just as a lame duck and loser: The care receiver occupies another position and wants to been seen in that respect);
- sealing and stabilizing the given recognition into a reliable resource (being faithful and not leaving).

### *C. Hermeneutical*

The third dimension of tuning is hermeneutical, being concerned with the interpretation of care needs. Some potential care receivers ask explicit questions (which need to be interpreted too) but in many cases there is no explicit question or demand. People *show* their life, their pain, their dreams, their pride, their boundaries, and it is up to care givers to understand what would be appropriate care, what is asked, desired, what the moral appeal is, what is missing. Here the emphasis is not on "accepting" the appeal (see above) but on interpreting it. One has to find and interpret the signs and check the interpretation. The meaning of a wish or yearning may change on a daily basis, and the tendency in care to say, "We should determine what is needed and from that fixed finding go on in providing care," is a fallacy. There is seldom anything like a stable and unambiguous (interpretation of) need. Getting acquainted with the need is not a unique phase in the process of caring; the interpretation of care-need requires ceaseless checking, and correction as necessary. There will never be quiet certainty in the care giver's mind about what, indisputably, is needed.

### *D. Critical*

Finally, the fourth dimension of tuning is of an (ideological-) critical nature. Understanding needs, and drawing on that understanding to provide care, does not happen in isolation, but in the highly complex zone of interference between the system and real life. Intertwined categorical and the institutional discourses apply, as do law and personal freedom, market discipline and compassionate humanity. This is obvious, but we must not forget that tuning is more than a technical, phenomenological and hermeneutic operation. The required art is to avoid naivety and innocence on the one hand and excessive sternness on the other. The determination of needs and appropriate care are operations under huge (cultural and systemic) pressure and are subject to "pollution" by interests that have nothing to do with good care. Awareness of how "stowaways" (interfering, hidden interests) get aboard processes of care giving is crucial. The presence of such stowaways is the rule rather than the exception: systemic logics, hardly controllable (institutional) dynamics, the quest for political profit, personal ambitions, false promises, unmanageable feelings of professional powerlessness and revulsion, all come with the care giving enterprise. Ideological-critical analysis is preferable to pious pronouncements when it comes to confronting hidden interests in care giving.

## 3. Efficacy

The key to the next criterion of "good care" is the question: Does it work? Has it the intended good results? Whereas "tuning" is internally linked to the "relevance" of care, "efficacy" is related to "truth." Care must, so to speak, deliver what it promises: it must be reliable, trustworthy, accurate. It must meet its claim to help and to care: it must be true. Efficacy has three dimensions.

### *A. Groundedness*

Today more than ever, the claim to efficacy (of the care to be provided) must be plausible. Everywhere the magic word is "evidence based practices," meaning that one should only allow / finance those methods and approaches that have been tested and had their effectiveness proved. Care practices should be "evidence based." No matter how obvious this call for "evidence based practices" may seem, recent discussions have shown the insufficiencies of the doctrine. Out of all the criticism, we will single out two objections (Vosman & Baart 2008). (i) The efficacy of social *practices* such as care is extraordinarily complex and disorderly. The claim to be able to identify and isolate a handful of variables that contribute decisively to good results, to assert their general validity and impose them deductively upon new practices, goes too far. The compulsory statistical procedures are an impediment, because of their *analytic* character. (ii) A second objection concerns the *nature* of the helpful knowledge. Evidence-based practices are rooted in a specific relation of practice to theory, where the practice has no wisdom of its own and consists of the application of "true" theory and "statistically significant" regularities. Local validation, contextual fine-tuning, tacit knowledge, practical and moral wisdom and ongoing learning processes in the execution of the care, are too easily disregarded. Nobody will seriously turn up their nose at "evidence-based practices" but to achieve good care we need more than that. Let us briefly point out some alternatives or supplements. The required *groundedness* is also realized in the just-mentioned local validation and continuously reflective learning. Some would say we need case-based learning, and management systems that encourage such "learning communities of practitioners" or "communities of practice." Besides endorsing "evidence based practices," one should promote "practice-based evidence," and make more room for the so-called "tacit knowledge" of practitioners' clinical wisdom and experienced intuition. The careful distillation of practical wisdom and the sharing of its (restricted) technical validity and moral desirability in a community of practice, contribute seriously to the groundedness of professional knowledge.

Or, at least, the application of regular evidence based knowledge should be wise—wisdom encompasses evidence and regulates its use.

Accountability is more than the redemption of the professional claim (we will do such and such, and it will "work"). It is also the inquiry into the so-called "experienced benefit" on the part of the care receiver: the professional claim and client's experience do not necessarily match. Lastly, groundedness also depends on the "plasticity" of the offered methods and knowledge, their adjustability and readiness to be made "consonant" with local life worlds, cultures, value systems, etc.

### *B. Performance*

Good care is care that is well *performed* or provided: there is no need to illustrate this proposition, although one can also imagine poor performance with good outcomes. The crucial component in "good performance" will undoubtedly be "competence"—and that competence will be related to the "groundedness" of the chosen approach. All this may be self-evident and in no need of elaboration. But allow us to add three simple criteria of good performance.

- As mentioned before, competent professionalism is currently associated with "obedience": a modern professional is characterized by their adherence to rules, agreements, procedures, scientific insights and bureaucratic reasoning. But practical evidence shows that competent care givers are also *capable of leaving the rules out and violating procedures*. In such cases, the preferable response is not punishment but education, by which one learns when to stick to the rules and when (and how) to sensibly abandon them. This supposes the professional is more than a domesticated monkey or an inanimate instrument in the hands of extra-situational forces. The ability to trespass in a sensible way presupposes (the acquirement of) virtues, such as prudence, discernment and "epikeia"—all carefully explored by Frans Vosman (1997; 2001 and 2008 with Baart; see also: Crève 1948 and Hibbs 2001).
- A second criterion of good performance is *discretion*. Good performance exceeds the social technical abilities and claims "discretional room," or autonomy to decide on the basis of one's own (professional) insights and skills. Here, more is at stake than the *right* to decide by oneself; the crux of the matter is the *moral agency* of one's own behaviour. To put it bluntly, it is useless to appoint workers with highly refined skills and concomitantly to foil decisions rooted in that capacity (Weggeman 2000; 2007). Or, to put it another way: What are we doing to care givers and other helpers if we deny their (own) moral experiences and competence?
- Thirdly, we must add the "*personal factor*" or "the person of the caregiver" to our answer to the question of what constitutes "good performance." By that we mean more than the "human person" behind the care giver in his or her role; we also refer to the necessity that a good carer understands something of his / her own life, feelings, fate, preferences, character etc. The ability to engage in mature introspection and solid reflection is indispensable, at least in avoiding the projection and the transfer of feelings to the care-receiver.

### C. Effect

The last dimension of efficacy concerns the *effects* of care. Because of the specific character of care, as explained above, our attention is not solely on efficiency but (also) on results and effects. Four points are especially relevant here.

- Good effects should be *proportional*, which means they should be reasonable when it comes to the price paid by the care receiver. One may pay the price in money but also by accepting humiliation, distrust and maltreatment, by slavishly filling in dozens of forms and repeating one's questions endlessly or by satisfying oneself with help that was not asked for but was the only one that could be delivered. The efforts of the care giver are not calculated here; of course he does not find himself in a dependent position and may put an end to an investment that is becoming too expensive. Nevertheless the price may also become too high for him to pay, e.g. when he is beaten up, threatened or risks suffering from burn-out or "compassion fatigue." (We come back to this below). Undesired side-effects raise the price for the care-receiver.
- As already said, good effects of care are always effects that are —immediately, in the long run, or retrospectively—*experienced* as good by the care-receiver (Tronto 1993; Van Heijst 2001; 2002; 2008a). It is indefensible to say the effects of care are good, but patients, the poor, or the homeless cannot feel their goodness. Asking for feedback, therefore, is an essential regulating principle of good care. One who does not seriously look to see what benefit is experienced as a result of his care does not care at all.
- We need to emphasise in this context the classic distinction between "outcomes" and "effects." An outcome is the result of care and the effect is the way that result makes itself felt in the longer run, as a lasting carry-over. If I want to help immigrants learn our language, I may report at the end of the year the *results* or *outcomes*:

12 women have attended the weekly lessons on a primary level and only two of them have dropped out. We may be satisfied to learn this, but these *results* don't inform us about the *effects* of the lessons. Do the women speak our language sufficiently or, more importantly, are they capable of getting along? The same is true when providing care. Ultimately we should not be interested in how much food and medicine is distributed, how many orphans are taken in or how many houses are built. The more important question is: What is the effect of all this in the long run, and what effect do we / they want? This kind of question is highly relevant to the care of frail elderly people and of youngsters with behavioral problems living in homes; the frequently heard complaint is that they are cared for but nobody is looking after them. Were we to believe the figures of the applicable quality systems, care couldn't be better.

- Finally, a word about a criterion we choose *not* to include. It is usual to add to a list like this one the criterion: good effects are effects "*as meant.*" According to this (rejected) criterion, if we make huge efforts to care for the hungry, we should not be satisfied if in the end we gave them blankets but did not feed them. Blankets may be a good result, but they are not the result *as meant*. What we intended to do has not been done, so we must be critical of the quality of our care. This criterion calls for the avoidance of *side-steps*, warning of the temptation to flee to another, easier target when the original target proves difficult to reach. The criterion also pays attention to how translations into professional language and applications of professional "diagnoses" can result in the step-by-step distortion or loss of the original question. People may receive help and appreciate what is done, but on closer inspection the results turn out to be largely unrelated to their original needs. The "distortion" is due to common professional procedures and institutional segmentation. The professional regime has difficulty handling disorderly needs. In short, good results should be "as meant." Nevertheless, we reject this criterion. We brought forward the idea that needs may change, become gradually clearer, and show themselves gradually in a trusting relationship developed over a long period of time: accordingly, we may not stick to the criterion "as meant." Our earlier criterion presupposes that anything like "the original question," anything fixed that precisely and frozen, should be avoided. Having said that, the rejected criterion provides a useful critical question to ask about so-called good results: How do they relate to the starting point of the care process?

## 4. Legitimacy

What makes care good care? Our response thus far has been:

1 It must have the proper identity: it must actually *be* care;
2 It must be relevant: fine-tuned to the specified needs;
3 It must be true, that is, effective.

Let us now turn to the fourth criterion: Good care must be *legitimate*. We will sketch four dimensions of legitimacy: care should be virtuous, decent, social and respectful. Although each of these dimensions deserves an extensive (political-ethical) treatise, we will be brief.

### *A. Virtuous*

Care should be morally sound and defensible, and, in principle, legal. We should consider the legitimacy of means (such as the use of unauthorized force or violence) and ends (for example, purposely ending human life or sterilizing mentally disabled people). But that is not enough. Depending on culture and context, some "illegitimate" actions are not illegal at all or may be executed under the strict condition that the all criteria of carefulness are meticulously and openly met. Our plea is for legitimacy understood not according to "legality" but rather according to "virtuousness." Good care should in principle not violate the law, but there may be instances which good care can be given only in violation of the law (just as good care may require the setting aside of professional rules, *supra*). Sometimes the law is unreasonable or not subtle enough to provide an adequate answer to a problem, i.e. (in our country) the fate of refugees and people asking for asylum. There may be times when the urgency is so high that one has hardly any choice but to go out and steal (medicine, bread, fuel). As a matter of fact, Catholic moral law doesn't forbid stealing in such emergency cases. The criterion boils down to this: Care must be *morally sound*. It must be defensible on the grounds that it is just and is done according to justifiable motives by virtuous carers. The morality of the care has reference not to a proclaimed and undoubted set of prescriptions, but instead to a richer reference frame that takes in traditional views, experience and intuition together, with everything being open to discussion and disputation. We are talking about the moral education of the carer, about discourse ethics and moral decisions made within a social community (as opposed to *in abstracto* reference to holy principles and duties).

### *B. Decent*

Apart from the legal and moral foundations of care, legitimacy also refers to the nature of the treatment. Good care does not humiliate (Margalit 1996; Sennett 2003) the care seeker. In practice, though, we find hundreds of examples to the contrary. People are met with constant suspicion, humbled by the administrative machinery, treated as "human flesh with a disease," abased through denial of their social-cultural position, honor or obligations. They are forced to wait unnecessarily, undress in the front of their children, asked to present official papers (such as birth certificates) when those in charge know they no longer exist, and so on. All these things happen in the process of getting the care one needs. Ironically, these violations of "human dignity" take place within the bounds of law and rights: The provision of care is regulated, restricted and tied to specific conditions, with much humiliation resulting from investigation into whether compulsory conditions have been fulfilled so that care may be provided. Here "claiming your rights" goes hand-in-hand with the loss of self-respect and self-esteem. That is why we have to add the criterion of personal, political and institutional *decency* to that of virtuousness within the framework of legitimacy.

### C. Social

Care, as mentioned before, is not given in a societal vacuum. On the contrary, society as such and politicians in particular bring intentions and expectations to the matter of care giving, its institutions and its funding. For example, they want to stop poverty, to remove homeless people from public space, or to bring domestic violence to an end. They want the dying to die decently in hospices and mothers to have the opportunity to care for their children. Legitimate care cannot ignore such expectations, and it is true that a considerable amount of care has originated from such measures. But again, we should not adhere slavishly to socio-political mandates. Take for example the actual Dutch policy on homeless people (most of whom are psychiatric patients, addicts, irreversibly (brain) damaged and unable to run their life properly). Whereas the emphasis used to lie with shelter, food and hygiene ("bed, bread and bath"), on safe havens, health care and social reintegration, today the problem is typically conceptualized as a matter of intolerable social inconvenience that must be combatted. The choice of words does not differ from programs to destroy rats, mice and other vermin—being merciless, determined and undeterred by consideration or empathy. Right-wing and left-wing politicians sense electoral profit and opportunity. Care for the homeless is affected by this "change of societal paradigm" and is arranged mainly to alleviate disturbance of the well-to-do ("the right not to be disturbed"), rather than to provide affectionate care to the least amongst us. Legitimate care in this context, however, does not mean blind obedience, but long-lasting concentration on social cohesion. When possible, care helps people to be respected and useful members of the community, rather than expelling them from the community. The social dimension of legitimate care supersedes political trends and has—its own basic social values available for corrective purposes. Good care doesn't deny its inherent political dimension and participates in the public debate on its objectives and values —more than ever necessary in our country! As is stated in the presence approach: *Being present with* the care receivers entails the obligation *to make present* their needs on another aggregative level, be it within management circles, in a political context, or on the university campus, etc. Forgetfulness is a form of unfaithfulness.

### D. Respectful

Legitimate care respects the personal integrity of the care receiver. Integrity (Musschenga 2004) is a complex and much disputed concept, but for the moment we will restrict its meaning to whatever can be combined with one's identity, selfhood and the personal ability to bear. If one's integrity is disrespected, one's boundaries are violated, one is alienated from oneself, and the (bodily or moral) coherence of one's life is affected. Even when the care offered is just, lawful, decent and socially acceptable, it stops being legitimate care if the receiver does not actually want it, cannot receive or bear it or is unable to integrate it in his life. Of course one may enter into conversation with recalcitrant care receivers, when serious effects may result from the rejection of care (by refusing to take medicine, undergo medical examination, eat properly, etc.). The care giver has an undeniable responsibility, which is sometimes opposed to that of the care receiver (Van der Lans et al. 2003). Good care has, when necessary, no aversion to dispute or quarrel. It is a misconception to think of care as something easy, lovely or romantic. In care, quality of life is at stake and is worth fighting for (Baart 2002b). But even in such circumstances, there is a bottom line of respect, autonomy and personal integrity. In care, the care receiver has the last word, not the care giver. A good care giver knows when to stop and is capable of allowing things to take their course. The most complicated cases are those in which the person in need of care is—temporarily or definitely— not accountable or beyond reach. The right to be respected, also in their autonomy, does not expire in such situations (Sennett 2003). In our country we have (methodological, political and moral) discussions on the so called "worrisome care escapist" (in Dutch: *zorgwekkende zorgmijder*): someone terribly in need of care but constantly running away from the care provided and avoiding every contact with care-givers (for instance, homeless, addicted, lonesome and psychiatrically disturbed tramps).

In order to decide which care may be given, another party should step in and stand for the interests of the unaccountable; that party may be the law, a close family member, a guardian or someone else, *as long as this agency takes the stance of befriendment*. The friend cares for the good of the other.

## 5. Feasibility

Good care is not only legitimate, effective and relevant; it is also doable. We do not have the necessary, technical aspects of performance foremost in mind here (the required strength, courage, understanding, means, time, money, facilities etc.), but two other related criteria. In this case, the focus on *feasibility* has to do with the care giver. Good care touches also the care giver.

### *A. Exhaustion*

To start with, this means that the carer should not be burned out by the care they are providing, nor should they become a victim of so-called "compassion fatigue."[3] Surprisingly, the burden of care experienced usually has little to do with the gravity of the problems the carer meets, be they matters of human suffering, death or injustice. Care givers can handle these serious problems if they are cared for themselves, especially if they receive that care in the course of their work. If their board of management is not really interested in their experience and always asking the wrong question (by fixating on calculable results, for example), or if their manager makes no allowance for their feelings (being too task-oriented), or if they are sent home without any serious debriefing (with their grief treated as a private and not a professional matter), then the equilibrium between investment and benefit becomes dangerously imbalanced, leading to burnout (*Werken aan balans* 2002). Similarly, when tiny results do not count (and only "solutions" are respected), when carers are not protected by their bosses from public attacks or legitimacy crises (with institutional pressure being passed on to individual collaborators), and when tasks are assigned without regard for individual talent, personality and limits, the risk of burn-out becomes all too real. Under such circumstances, caring becomes not do-able—not because of the work itself, but because of the organization's failure to adequately care for the carer.

### B. Responsiveness

Care for the caregiver includes the right of the carer to be *responsive*, up to and including the possibility of refusing duties, setting their own boundaries and indicating what morally they can handle. Good care givers are not only "empathic" but also socially combative and equipped with a healthy self-esteem. Good care can hardly be called care when the carer is unfeelingly coerced. If the agency is "hollowed out," not only is the accountable core removed from the care (that is, the human being who can be addressed, who can explain and, when necessary, justify what is offered or refused), but the opportunity for the carer to experience the care giving as personally meaningful is also ignored or devastated. The potential of the caregiver's self-fulfilment is eliminated from the caring process. The good of the process becomes external to the carer. That damages the feasibility of the care and is morally objectionable.

### Interlude 2: Recognition

Having so far explained from the perspective of the theory of presence how good care is identified, I now may formulate why I think care receivers have good reason to ask for recognition when care is provided or, to formulate it more precisely, recognition *in* the practice of care providing.

- Recognition in its threefold form[4] (emotional support, cognitive respect and social esteem, cf. Honneth) is an *affirmative* act and as such an act of *creation* and recreation of humans. Recognition absorbs the recognized one into social, public network relations and makes them meaningful and social. Because of this, care and recognition are logically interconnected.
- By recognition one's *inevitable vulnerability* is protected and so one's *dignity* and honorability are defended and humiliation is

prevented. Again, as with care, all recognition is internally linked up to vulnerability, be it constitutional, physical or social.
- Recognition confirms (and presupposes) one's *capacities, value and qualities* as a precious member of our society. And again, care does the same: It is useless to give care to something you believe should disappear because it is harmful, worthless or hopelessly lost.

Good care and recognition are thus tightly interwoven, without being identical or mutually exhaustive. In care if one really tries to include recognition, three conditions must be fulfilled: (1) The care giver should give up his self-referential (professional and personal) rights. (2) The care giver should choose a discourse in which the struggle for a mutual perspective may take place and the carer accepts being corrected. (3) The caregiver should be able to resist systemic pressure: the task to deal with reification procedures, interventionist logic and the organized struggle for recognition.

## 6. Mediation

As we bring this reflection to a close, we would like to focus—with some hesitation—on a fairly common criterion of good care. To our mind it is an intriguing hypothesis and well-founded proposal. Our starting point is simple: all care is mediated care. It is provided through (social) *relations*—a platitude, but a useful one, because those relations are *not just instrumental* to care provision but are, to a certain extent, the *care itself*. It is a misconception to assume that relations between the care giver and the care receiver are no more than vehicles for the transportation of caring acts and means. In reality, the most basic form of being cared for, a caring good in itself and *sui generis* (unique, not reducible to anything else) is embedded in relationships. Many pages in *Een theorie van de presentie* are spent explaining the blessings of being-in-relation, with the conclusion that people turn out to be happy and satisfied even when obvious problems are not solved. Apparently they are compensated by the fact that they are integrated within a meaningful relationship. The relationship is not instrumental nor strategically entered, but substantive and without need of something beyond itself to be fruitful, relieving and consoling. Of course, we are talking about good, social relations: If they lack this quality, they are not only not-good, they are something worse, being harmful and leading to abandonment and loneliness. That is the opposite of care.

The consequences of this insight are impressive. If all the other criteria are met (tuning, efficacy, legitimacy and feasibility), we may not yet be sure the care is of good quality: the embeddedness in strategic, instrumental intentions may yet corrupt the integrity of the relation and so lower the quality of care. Among professionals this requirement is not undisputed! Another consequence concerns management of the relationship, which involves the duty to ensure its moral soundness. If the care giver, in cooperation with the care receiver, does not succeed in managing the relationship in conformity to its purpose, the remaining transfer of care will also be blocked. Unsuccessful management of the relationship is recognizable by excess and derailment. Examples include sexual intercourse with the care receiver, hidden agendas, inappropriate nearness, projection and the transfer of one's own desires, silent interests, indecent intimacy, false hope, the lack of after-care etc. This criterion forces us to be alert to the dangers as well as the blessings of the so-called caring relationship.

The next consequence also touches upon the potential corruption of the relationship. If the integrity of the relationship is actually undermined by the "invisible hand" of the market, the bureaucracy and politics, one may wonder what kind of quality is realized. No evaluation of care should overlook the (barely traceable) network and powers in which care is provided. That influential embeddedness is, however, not necessarily restrictive: It may safeguard fairness, space and the accessibility of care.

In conclusion, we would like to suggest a question that draws on an earlier discussion of the presence approach. If care's quality is *a priori* dependent on the integrity of the relationship in which it is requested and provided, what does that mean for the witnesses of that care (and of that suffering, aspiration, etc.)? We would propose that those witnesses are *qualitate qua* and, strictly speaking, part of that relation and by consequence morally involved. They don't have the possibility of saying "I didn't know!" One might argue that, since they are not the carers themselves, they are not responsible for the care (and its quality). But this is a faulty argument. Witnesses are involved by virtue of their awareness. As such, they have the opportunity to heighten the quality of that care by reflecting publicly and with moral courage on what they have seen.

| ***Summary* What makes care good care?** | | |
|---|---|---|
| **Characteristics** | **Two interludes illustrating the internal links of good care and recognition** | **Explanation characteristics** |
| 1 It must have the proper identity. That is, it must actually *be* care. | | Good care is experienced *as* good care by the care receiver. |
| 2 It must be relevant, that is, fine-tuned to the specified needs. | | In four ways:<br>• Pragmatic avoiding mismatch<br>• Phenomenological → making room for the appeal<br>• Hermeneutical → interpreting the appeal<br>• Critical → avoiding naivety |

| | | |
|---|---|---|
| 3 It must be true, that is, effective. | | In three dimensions:<br>• Groundedness → it must work as promised and meant<br>• Performance → it must be done (morally) competently, including the handling of rules and one's own personality<br>• Effect → for a fair price and with a sound carry-over |
| 4 It must be legitimate in more respects than just legal. | | In four dimensions: care should be<br>• Virtuous<br>• Decent<br>• Social and<br>• Respectful |
| 5 It must be do-able, technically and humanly speaking. | | In two respects:<br>• Without exhaustion (burn-out or compassion fatigue)<br>• And with the possibility of refusing duties and trespassing the rules |
| 6 Good care is beneficence, a caring good in itself and *sui generis* | | The caring relation is ambiguous because of its social and systemic embeddedness. |

**Table 4: Summary of the answer on the question "What makes care good care"**

What makes care good care? Having summarized our findings (Table 4), we would add only the observation that care and social inclusion are identical. For that reason, the ethics of care requires a political and a moral program on behalf of human dignity, as much as it does social-scientific reconceptualization.

## Notes

[1] This text is based on Andries Baart (ed.), *Unheard stories of people infected and affected by hiv/aids about care and/or the lack of care*, special issue of *Sociale Interventie*, 13(2004)3 with his contribution: "What makes care good care?", 14-26.

[2] Besides the solid efforts made by Annelies van Heijst in her recent and less recent works to determine what care is or ought to be, we would like to mention Linus VanLaere (2006) and Jan Vorstenbosch (2005).

[3] "Compassion Fatigue is a state of tension and preoccupation with the individual or cumulative trauma of clients as manifested in one or more ways including re-experiencing the traumatic event, avoidance/numbing of reminders of the event, and persistent arousal. Although similar to critical incident stress (being traumatized by something you actually experience or see), with Compassion Fatigue you are absorbing the trauma through the eyes and ears of your clients. It can be thought of as secondary post-traumatic stress," so: http://www.ace-network.com/cfspotlight.htm#WhatIs%20CF (visited 21st Feb. 2009).

[4] Elaborated and criticized by Annelies van Heijst (2008b).

# LITERATURE


Adorno, Theodor W. 1983. *Prisms*. Cambridge, Mass: MIT Press.

Afshari, Reza. 2007. On Historiography of Human Rights: Reflections on Paul Gordon Lauren's "The Evolution of International Human Rights: Visions Seen". *Human Rights Quarterly* 29: 1-67.

Agich, George J. 2003. *Dependency and Autonomy in Old Age: An Ethical Framework for Long-Term Care*. Cambridge: Cambridge University Press.

Allmark, P. 1995. Can There Be an Ethics of Care? *Journal of Medical Ethics* 21: 19-24.

American Association on Intellectual and Developmental Disabilities. 2010. *The AAIDD Definition of Intellectual Disability*, http://www.aaidd.org

American Psychiatric Association. 2003. *Diagnostic and Statistical Manual of Mental Disorders*, Washington, American Psychiatric Association.

ANSA. 2008. *Italy 'To Curb Immigrant Influx'*. ANSA.it 2008 [cited 13 November 2008]. Available from http://www.ansa.it/site/notizie/awnplus/english/news/2008-11-13_113.

Arras, J. 1991. Getting down to cases: The revival of casuistry in bioethics. *Journal of Medicine and Philosophy* 16, 29-51.

Arras, J. 1997. Nice story, but so what? Narrative and justification in ethics. In *Stories and Their Limits*, ed. H. Nelson. New York: Routledge.

Austin, W., V. Bergum, J. Dossetor. 2003. Relational Ethics: An Action Ethic as a Foundation for Health Care. In *Approaches to Ethics: Nursing Beyond Boundaries*, ed. Verena Tschudin, 45-51. Edinburgh: Elsevier.

Baart, Andries. 2000. *Raken aan het geleefde leven*. 's-Hertogenbosch: Actioma.

Baart, Andries. 2001. *Een theorie van de presentie*. Utrecht: Lemma.

Baart, Andries. 2002a. *Aanzetten tot een theorie van de Derde Partij met behulp van de presentietheorie*. Den Haag: LCO.

Baart, Andries, Geert van der Laan. 2002b. Sociale interventie: koppeling van theorie en praktijk. *Sociale Interventie* 11 (4): 4-26.

Baart, Andries, Frans Vosman, eds. 2003a. *Present*. Utrecht: Lemma.

Baart, Andries, ed. 2003b. *Presentie* special issue of *Sociale Interventie* 12 (2).

Baart, Andries. 2004. *Aandacht. Etudes in presentie*. Utrecht: Lemma.

Baart, Andries. 2005. *Klein pleidooi tegen grote distantiëring in de zorg*, Utrecht.

Baart, Andries, Thijs Tromp, Annelies van Heijst. 2006a. *Minder hard—meer hart*. Utrecht.

Baart, Andries. 2006b. *Tweespraak. Vier gesprekken over het ene goed van presentie*. Utrecht.

Baart, Andries. 2006c. Leven en verlaten leven—over de betekenis van presentie voor vertrouwen. In *Congresverslag "Daar draait het allemaal om: presentie!"*. Utrecht: 4-16 (op: www.presentie.nl → Presentiecongres → Verslag).

Baart, Andries. 2007. *Kwetsbaar maar niet alleen kwetsbaar. Over het bereiken en steunen van multiproblem gezinnen, kwetsbare kinderen en tienermoeders*. Utrecht/ Den Bosch (2nd edition, also digital, 2008 → www.presentie.nl)

Baart, Andries. 2008a. *Kwetsbaarheid. Bemoeien. Regels—Drie Publiekslezingen aan de Universiteit van Tilburg najaar 2007* (box with three DVDs and a hand-out) Utrecht: Stichting Presentie.

Baart, Andries, Mieke Grypdonck. 2008b. *Verpleegkunde en presentie*. Den Haag: Lemma.

Baart, Andries, Frans Vosman. 2008c. Being witness to the lives of the very old. *Sociale Interventie* 17(3): 21-32.

Baier, Annette C. 1995. The Need for more than Justice. In *Justice and care. Essential readings in feminist ethics*, ed. Virgina Held, 47-60. Boulder, CO: Westview Press.

Bakhtin, M. 1981. Discourse in the Novel. In *The dialogic imagination*, ed. Michael Holquist (Caryl Emerson and Michael Holquist trans.). Austin: University of Texas Press.

Batson, C. D. et al. 1995. Immortality from empathy-induced altruism: when compassion and justice conflict. *Journal of Personality and Social Psychology* 68: 1042-54.

Benbassat J., R. Baumal. 2004. What is empathy, and how can it be promoted during clinical clerkships? *Academic Medicine* 79: 832-9.

Bertolami, C. N. 2004. Why our ethics curricula don't work. *Journal of Dental Education* 68: 414-25.

Bishop, A., J. Scudder. 1990. *The Practical, Moral and Personal Sense of Nursing: A Phenomenological Philosophy of Practice*. New York: State University of New York Press.

Bloom, S. W. 1989. The medical school as a social organization: the sources of resistance to change. *Medical Education* 23: 228-41.

Blum, L. 1980. *Friendship, Altruism and Morality*. London: Routledge.

Bohmeyer, Axel. 2008. Axel Honneths Theorie der Anerkennung. Feministische Bezüge und sozialethische Relevanz. In *Feministische Ethik und christliche Sozialethik*, ed. Christian Spieß and Katja Winkler, 253-76. Berlin.

Boleyn-Fitzgerald, P. 2003. Care and the problem of pity. *Bioethics* 17: 1-20.

Bolstanski, Luc. 1990. *L'Amour et la Justice comme compétences. Trois essais de sociologie de l'action*, Paris: Métailié.

Bouquez, N. 1997. *De beleving van patiënten met een cerebro-vasculair accident in de vroege periode van hun aandoening*. Licenciaatsscriptie Medisch-Sociale Wetenschappen, Universiteit Gent.

Boykin, A., S. Schoenhofer. 1993. *Nursing as Caring: A Model for Transforming Nursing*. New York: National League of Nursing Press.

Bubeck, D. E. 1995. *Care, Gender and Justice*. Oxford: Clarendon.

Buber, Martin. 1923. *Ich und Du*. Heidelberg: Schneider.

Butler, Judith. 1996. *Excitable Speech: A Politics of the Performative*. New York: Routledge.

Butler, Judith. 1990. *Gender Trouble: Feminism and the Subversion of Identity*, New York: Routledge.

Charmaz, K. 1991. *Good Days, Bad Days: The Self in Chronic Illness and Time*. New Brunswick, N.J.: Rutgers University Press.

Clapton, J. 2003. Tragedy and catastrophe: Contentious discourses of ethics and disability. *Journal of Intellectual Disability Research* 47 (7).

Collier, V.U. et al. 2002. Stress in medical residency: status quo after a decade of reform? *Annals of Internal Medicine* 136: 384-90.

Coulehan, J. 2005. Today's professionalism: Engaging the mind but not the heart. *Academic Medicine* 80: 892-8.

Corriere della Sera. 2008. *Green Light for 170,000 More Immigrants Priority for Home Helps and Carers* (Notizie di cronaca del Corriere della Sera), 8 November 2008 [cited 8 November 2008]. Available from http://www.corriere.it/english/08_noviembre_03/immigrants/_801538ee.

Covington, Holly. 2005. Caring presence. Providing a safe space for patients. *Holistic Nursing Practice* July/August : 169-72.

Crève, A. 1948. *De epikeia volgens Thomas van Aquino en Suarez*. Leuven (Series: *Sylloge excerptorum e dissertationibus ad gradum doctoris in sacra theologia vel in iure canonico consequendum conscriptis*; tom. 16, fasc. 4; reprinted from: *Miscellanea moralia in honorem Eximii Domini Arthur Janssen*, 1 (1948).

Crigger, N. J. 1997. The trouble with caring: A review of eight arguments against an ethic of care. *Journal of Professional Nursing* 13: 217-21.

Darwall, Stephen. 2006. *The Second-Person Standpoint: Morality, Respect, and Accountability*. Cambridge, Mass.: Harvard University Press.

Davis, A. J., Fowler, M. 2006. Caring and caring ethics depicted in selected literature: What we know and what we need to ask. In *Essentials of Teaching and Learning in Nursing Ethics: Perspectives and Methods*, ed. A. J. Davis, V. Tschudin, L. De Raeve, 165-79. Oxford: Elsevier.

DePaul, M. 1993. *Balance and Refinement: Beyond Coherence Methods of Moral Inquiry*. London: Routledge.

Derrida, J. 1970. Structure, sign and play in the discourse of the human sciences. In *The Languages of Criticism and the Sciences of Man: The Structuralist Controversy*, ed. R. Macksey and E. Donato. Baltimore: Johns Hopkins Press.

De Waal, F. 2001. *Good Natured. The Origins of Right and Wrong in Humans and Other Animals*. Cambridge (Mass.): Harvard University Press.

De Waal, F. 2006. Morally evolved. Primate social instincts, human morality, and the rise and fall of 'Veneer Theory'. In *Primates and Philosophers: How Morality Evolved*, ed. F. De Waal, 1-82. Princeton/Oxford: Princeton University Press.

Dewettinck, I., M. Grypdonck, A. Dhondt. 2001. Leven met vochtbeperking: een moeilijke opdracht. *TVZ. Tijdschrift voor Verpleegkundigen*: 675-80.

Diggins, K. 2007. Compassion or pity? *J Christ. Nurs* 24: 81.

Dinsmore, C. E., S. Daugherty, H. J. Zeitz. 2001. Student responses to the gross anatomy laboratory in a medical curriculum. *Clinical Anatomy* 14: 231-6.

Dubet, Francois. 2002. *Le Déclin de l'institution*, Paris: Seuil.

Duprez, V., M. Grypdonck. 2002. Therapietrouw bij chronisch zieken die in armoede leven. *TVZ. Tijdschrift voor Verpleegkundigen* 112: 62-5.

Eikeland, Olav. 2008. *The Ways of Aristotle. Aristotelian Phronesis, Aristotelian Philosophy of Dialogue, and Action Research*. Berlin etc.: Peter Lang.

Erikson, E. 1964. *Insight and Responsibility. Lectures on the Ethical Implications of Psychoanalytic Insight*. New York: Norton.

Ferry, Jean-Marc. 1991. *Les puissances de l'expérience*. Tome II: *Les ordres de la reconnaissance*, Paris : Cerf.

Fingeld-Connett, Deborah. 2006. Meta-synthesis of presence in nursing. *Journal of Advanced Nursing* 55(6): 708-14.

Fingeld-Connett, Deborah. 2007. Meta-synthesis of caring in Nursing. *Journal of Clinical Nursing* 17: 196-204.

Fisher, Berenice, Joan Tronto. 1990. Toward a feminist theory of caring. In *Circles of Care: Work and Identity in Women's Lives*, ed. E. K. Abel, M. K. Nelson, 35-62. Albany, N.Y.: State University of New York Press.

Fogerty, L. A., et al. 1999. Can 40 seconds of compassion reduce patient anxiety? *Journal of Clinical Oncology* 17(1): 371-9.

Frankfurt, H. G. 2004. *The Reasons of Love*. Princeton NJ/Oxford: Princeton University Press.

Frankl, V. E. 1963. *Man's Search for Meaning: An Introduction to Logotherapy*. New York: Washington Square Press.

Fraser, Nancy. 1997. *Justice Interruptus: Critical Reflections on the "Postsocialist" Condition*. New York/London: Routledge.

Fraser, Nancy & Axel Honneth. 2003. *Redistribution or Recognition: A Political-Philosophical Exchange*, London/New York.

Fraser, Nancy. 2005. Mapping the feminist imagination: From redistribution to recognition to representation. *Constellations: An International Journal of Critical & Democratic Theory* 12 (3): 295-307.

Fredriksson, L., K. Eriksson. 2003. The ethics of the caring conversation. *Nursing Ethics* 10: 138-48.

Friedlaender, G. 2006. The 80-hour duty week. Rationale, early attitudes, and future questions, *Clinical Orthopaedics and Related Research* 449: 138-42.

Gadow, S. A. 1985. Nurse and patient: The caring relationship. In *Caring, Curing, Coping*, ed. A. H. Bishop and J. R. Scudder, 31-43. Birmingham AL: University of Alabama Press.

Gastmans, Chris, B. Dierckx de Casterlé, P. Schotsmans. 1998. Nursing considered as moral practice: A philosophical-ethical interpretation of nursing. *Kennedy Institute of Ethics Journal* 8: 43-69.

Gastmans, Chris & Linus Vanlaere. 2005. *Cirkels van zorg. Ethisch omgaan met ouderen*, Leuven.

Gastmans, Chris & Kris Dierickx, eds. 2006. *Ethiek in witte jas. Zorgzaam omgaan met het leven*. Leuven: Davidsfonds.

Gaul, A. L. 1995. Casuistry, care, compassion, and ethics data analysis. *Advances in Nursing Science* 17(3): 47-57.

Gilligan, Carol. 1982. *In a Different Voice: Psychological Theory and Women's Development*. Cambridge MA/London: Harvard University Press.

Gilligan, Carol. 1995. Moral orientation and moral development, in *Justice and Care. Essential Readings in Feminist Ethics*, ed. Virgina Held, 31-47. Boulder, CO: Westview Press.

Glasberg, A., S. Eriksson, A. Norberg. 2007. Burnout and stress of conscience among healthcare personnel. *Journal of Advanced Nursing* 57: 392-403.

Glenn, E. N. 2000. Creating a caring society. *Contemporary Sociology* 29: 84-95.

Goodin, Robert E. 1985. *Protecting the Vulnerable: A Reanalysis of Our Social Responsibilities*. Chicago: University of Chicago Press.

Goodrich, Joanna, Jocelyn Cornwell. 2008. *Seeing the Person in the Patient*, London: The King's Fund.

Green, Donald, Ian Shapiro. 1994. *Pathologies of Rational Choice Theory*. New Haven: Yale University Press.

Greenspan, S. 1999. What is meant by mental retardation? *International Review of Psychiatry* 11: 6-18.

Griffin, A. P. 1983. A Philosophical analysis of caring in nursing. *Journal of Advanced Nursing* 8: 289-95.

Grypdonck, Mieke. 2002. *Palliatieve zorg, zorg voor het leven*, Leuven.

Grypdonck, Mieke, S. Weldam, M. J. Litjens. 2003. *Richtlijn ter bevordering van adequaat zelfmanagement bij hemodialysepatiënten met betrekking tot de vochtbeperking, een behoeftegestuurde benadering*. Disciplinegroep Verplegingswetenschap, Universiteit Utrecht. Utrecht: UMCUtrecht

Grypdonck, Mieke. 2005. *Tussen verpleegkunde en* verplegingswetenschap. Utrecht: UMCUtrecht.

Habermas, Jürgen. 1990. Justice and solidarity. On the discussion concerning stage 6. In *The Moral Domain. Essays in the Ongoing Discussion between Philosophy and the Social Sciences*, ed. Thomas E. Wren. Cambridge, Mass.: MIT Press.

Habermas, Jürgen. 1991. *Justification and Application: Remarks on Discourse Ethics*. Cambridge, Mass: MIT Press.

Habermas, Jürgen. 1995. *Moral Consciousness and Communicative Action*. Cambridge, Mass.: MIT Press.

Hafferty, F. H., R. Franks. 1994. The hidden curriculum, ethics teaching, and the structure of medical education. *Academic Medicine* 69: 861-71.

Halpern J. 2003. What is clinical empathy? *Journal of General Internal Medicine* 18: 670-4.

Hawkesworth, Mary. 2006. *Feminist Inquiry: From Political Conviction to Methodological Innovation*. New Brunswick, NJ: Rutgers University Press.

Hawkins, A. H. 1997. Medical ethics and the epiphanic dimension of narrative. In *Stories and their Limits*, ed. H. Nelson. New York: Routledge.

Hertogh, C. 2004. Ethiek van de zorg voor ouderen met dementie: De positie van verzorgenden. [Care ethics for older persons with dementia: The position of carers]. *Denkbeeld. Tijdschrift voor Psychogeriatrie [Journal of Psychogeriatrics]*. August: 2-8.

Heymann, Jody. 2000. *The Widening Gap: Why America's Working Families Are in Jeopardy and What Can Be Done About It.* New York: Basic.

Hibbs, Thomas S. 2001. *Virtue's Splendor: Wisdom, Prudence, and the Human Good*, New York: Fordham University Press (Series: Moral Philosophy and Moral Theology: no. 3).

Hoare, C. H. 2002. *Erikson and Development in Adulthood: New Insights from the Unpublished Papers.* Oxford/New York: Oxford University Press.

Honneth, Axel. 1992 (erweiterte Ausgabe 2003). *Kampf um Anerkennung: Zur moralischen Grammatik sozialer Konflikte.* Frankfurt am Main.

Honneth, Axel. 1995a. *The Struggle for Recognition: The Moral Grammar of Social Conflicts.* Cambridge, Mass.: MIT Press. [translation of *Kampf der Anerkennung*]

Honneth, Axel. 1995b. The other of justice. Habermas and the ethical challenge of postmodernism. In *The Cambridge Companion to Habermas*, ed. Stephen K. White, 289-323. New York: Cambridge University Press.

Honneth, Axel. 2000. *Das Andere der Gerechtigkeit.* Frankfurt am Main.

Honneth, Axel & Nancy Fraser. 2003. *Redistribution or Recognition? A Political-Philosophical Exchange.* London/New York: Verso.

Honneth, Axel. 2005a. *Reification: A Recognition-Theoretical View.* The Tanner Lectures on Human Values. Delivered at University of California, Berkeley, March 14-16, 2005 [accessible: http://www.tannerlectures.utah.edu/lectures/documents/Honneth_2006.pdf]

Honneth, Axel. 2005b. *Verdinglichung: Eine anerkennungstheoretische Studie.* Frankfurt am Main.

Honneth, Axel. 2005c. Between Aristotle and Kant – Sketch of a morality of recognition. *Advances in Psychology* 137 ("Morality in Context"): 41-56.

Honneth, Axel & Joel Anderson. 2005. Autonomy, vulnerability, recognition, and justice. In *Autonomy and the Challenges to Liberalism*, ed. J. Anderson and A. Christman, 127-49. New York: Cambridge University Press.

Honneth, Axel. 2007a. The other of justice: Habermas and the ethical challenge of postmodernism. In *Disrespect. The Normative Foundations of Critical Theory.* Cambridge: Polity Press, 99-128. [Translation of *Das Andere der Gerechtigkeit*]

Honneth, Axel. 2007b. Love and morality: On the moral content of emotional ties. In *Disrespect.* Cambridge: Polity Press.

Honneth, Axel. 2008. *Reification. A New Look at an Old Idea.* Oxford: Oxford University Press.

Hoover, J. 2002. The personal and professional impact of undertaking an educational module on human caring. *Journal of Advanced Nursing* 37: 79-86.

Housset, Emmanuel. 2003. *L'intelligence de la pitié: Phénoménologie de la communauté.* Paris: Cerf.

Huggard, P. 2003. Compassion fatigue: how much can I give? *Medical Education* 37: 163-4.

Hunnert, E. M., F. Hafferty, D. Christakis. 1996. Characteristics of the informal curriculum and trainee's ethical choices. *Academic Medicine* 71: 624-33.

Jameson, F. 1974. *The Prison-House of Language: A Critical Account of Structuralism and Russian Formalism*. Princeton: Princeton University Press.

Janssens, Louis. 1972. Ontic evil and moral evil. *Louvain Studies* 4; 115-56.

Jecker, N. S., D. J. Self. 1991. Separating care and cure: An analysis of historical and contemporary images of nursing and medicine. *The Journal of Medicine and Philosophy* 16: 285-306.

Jecker, N. S., W. Reich. 2004. Contemporary Ethics of Care. In *Encyclopedia of Bioethics*, ed. S. Post. New York: Thomson & Gale.

Johnson, A., S. Toulmin. 1988. *The Abuse of Casuistry*. Berkeley and Los Angeles: University of California Press.

Kars, Marijke, Mieke Grypdonck, Maria De Korte-Verhoef, Willem Kamps, Esther Meijer-van den Bergh, Marian Verkerk, Johannes van Delden. 2009. Parental experience at the end-of-Life in children with cancer: 'Preservation' and 'letting go' in relation to loss, *Supportive Care in Cancer*.

King, N., C. Carroll, P. Newton, T. Dornan. 2002. You can't cure it so you have to endure it: the experience of adaptation to diabetic renal disease. *Qualitative Health Research* 12: 329-46.

Kittay, Eva Feder. 1999. *Love's Labor: Essays on Women, Equality, and Dependency*. New York: Routledge.

Kittay, Eva Feder. 2002. When caring is just and justice is caring. In *The Subject of Care: Feminist Perspectives on Dependency*, ed. Eva Feder Kittay and Ellen K. Feder. New York: Rowman & Littlefield.

Kittay, Eva Feder. 2003. Disability, equal dignity and care. *Concilium* 39: 105-15.

Kittay, Eva Feder. 2009. Ideal theory bioethics and the exclusion of people with severe cognitive disabilities. In *Naturalized Bioethics: Responsible Knowing and Practice*, ed. Marian Verkerk, Hilde Lindemann and Margaret Urban Walker, 218-37. New York: Cambridge University Press.

Kittay, Eva Feder. 2005. At the margins of personhood. *Ethics* 116: 100-31.

Kojève, Alexandre. 1980. *Introduction to the Reading of Hegel*. Ithaca: Cornell University Press.

Korsgaard, Christine. 1996. *Creating the Kingdom of Ends*. Cambridge, Mass.: Cambridge University Press.

Krebs, D., M. Janicki. 2004. Biological foundations of moral norms. In *The Psychological Foundations of Culture*, ed. M. Schaller, C. S. Crandall, 125-48. Mahwah NJ/London: Lawrence Erlbaum Associates.

Kunneman, Harry. 2005. *Voorbij het dikke ik. Bouwstenen voor een kritisch humanisme*. Amsterdam.

Kymlicka, Will. 1994. *Multicultural Citizenship*. Oxford: Oxford University Press.

Lauren, Paul Gordon. 2003. *The Evolution of International Human Rights: Visions Seen*. Philadelphia: University of Pennsylvania Press.

Leget, Carlo. 2003. *Ruimte om te sterven. Een weg voor zieken, naasten en zorgverleners*. Tielt: Lannoo.

Leget, Carlo. 2004. Avoiding evasion: medical ethics education and emotion theory. *Journal of Medical Ethics* 30; 490-3.

Leget, Carlo, Gert Olthuis. 2005. Compassie & Co. Medelijden als basis van morele vorming en de kansen van portfolio-onderwijs. *Tijdschrift voor Gezondheidszorg en Ethiek* 15: 106-11.

Leget, Carlo, Gert Olthuis. 2007. Compassion as a basis for ethics in medical education. *Journal of Medical Ethics* 33: 617-20.

Leira, A. 1994. Concepts of caring: Loving, thinking, and doing. *Social Service Review* 62: 185-201.

Letiche, Hugo. 2008. *Making Healthcare Care*. Charlotte NC.: IAP.

Liégeois, Axel. 2005. Ethical dilemmas in community mental health care. *Journal of Medical Ethics* 31 (8): 452-6.

Liégeois, Axel, M. Eneman. 2008. An ethics of deliberation, consent and coercion in psychiatry. *Journal of Medical Ethics* 34 (2): 73-6.

Liégeois, Axel. 2009. *Waarden in dialoog. Ethiek in de zorg*. Leuven: LannooCampus.

Lindemann, K. 2003. The ethics of receiving. *Theoretical Medicine and Bioethics* 24: 501-9.

Little, M.O. 1998. Care. From theory to orientation and back. *Journal of Medicine and Philosophy* 23: 190-209.

Logghe, A., J. Peeters. 2006. *Therapie(on)trouw bij diabetes melitus patiënten*. Medisch-Sociale Wetenschappen, Universiteit Gent.

MacIntyre, Alisdair. 1984. *After Virtue*. Notre Dame: University of Notre Dame Press.

MacIntyre, Alisdair. 1988. *Whose Justice? Which Rationality?* Notre Dame: University of Notre Dame Press.

Mangione S., et al. 2002. Assessment of empathy in different years of internal medicine training. *Medical Teacher* 24: 370-3.

Manschot, Henk and Marian Verkerk ed. 1994. *Ethiek van de zorg: Een discussie*. Amsterdam, Meppel.

Margalit, Avishai. 1996. *The Decent Society*. Cambridge, MA: Harvard University Press (translated from the Hebrew by Naomi Goldblum).

Maslow, Abraham H. 1999. *Toward a Psychology of Being*. New York: Wiley (3th edition; foreword and ed.: Richard Lowry).

May, R. 1969. *Love and Will*. New York: Norton.

Mayeroff, M. 1971. *On Caring*. New York: Harper & Row.

McCance, T. V., H. P. McKenna, J. R. P. Boore. 1997. Caring: dealing with a difficult concept. *International Journal for Nursing Studies* 34: 241-8.

*Measuring Program Outcomes: A Practical Approach*. 1996. Alexandria, VA: United Way of America.

Mead, George Herbert. 1934. *Mind, Self and Society from the Standpoint of a Social Behaviorist*. Chicago: Chicago University Press.

Medical School Objectives Writing Group. 1999. Learning objectives for medical student education-guidelines for medical schools: report I of the Medical School Objectives Project. *Academic Medicine* 74: 13-8.

Melief, Willem. 2003. Evidence-based practice in sociale interventies. *Sociale Interventie* 12 (4): 17-29.

Meyers, Diana Tietjens ed. 1997. *Feminist Social Thought: A Reader*. New York [especially: Care and its Critics, 547-692].

Mittal V., E. D. Portnier. 2006. Continuity of care in the 80-hour workweek era? *Current Surgery* 23: 31-4.

Morse, J. M., S. M. Solberg, W. L. Neander, J. L. Bottorff, J. L. Johnson. 1990. Concepts of caring and caring as concept. *Advances in Nursing Science* 13: 1-14.

Morse, J. M., J. L. Bottorff, W. L. Neander, S. M. Solberg. 1991. Comparative analysis of conceptualizations and theories of caring. *Journal of Nursing Scholarship* 23: 119-26.

Musschenga, Bert. 2004. *Integriteit. Eenheid en heelheid van de mens*, Utrecht: Lemma.

Nelson, H. L. 1992. Against caring. *The Journal of Clinical Ethics* 3: 8-30.

Nelson, H. L. 2001. *Damaged Identities, Narrative Repair*. Ithaca NY: Cornell University Press.

Nelson, H. L. ed. 1997. *Stories and their Limits: Narrative Approaches to Bioethics*. New York: Routledge.

Nickel, James. 2005. Poverty and rights. *The Philosophical Quarterly* 55: 385-402.

Nietzsche, Friedrich. 1878. *Human, all too Human* (Ger: *Menschliches, Allzumenschliches*), trans. Gary Handwerk, Stanford University Press, 1997.

Nietzsche, Friedrich. 1881. *Daybreak* (Ger: *Aurora*), trans. R. J. Hollingdale, Cambridge University Press, 1997.

Nietzsche, Friedrich. 1882. *The Gay Science* (Ger: *Die fröhliche Wissenschaft*) ed. Bernard Williams, trans. Josefine Nauckhoff and Adrian Del Caro, Cambridge University Press, 2001.

Nietzsche, Friedrich. 1886. *Beyond Good and Evil* (Ger: *Jenseits von Gut und Böse*) trans. Judith Norman, Cambridge University Press, 2001.

Nietzsche, Friedrich. 1901. *Posthumous Fragments (The Will to Power; Ger; Der Wille zur Macht), trans. W. Kaufmann* and R. J.. Hollingdale (New York: *Vintage* Books, *1968)*.

Noddings, Nel. 1984. *Caring: Feminine Approach to Ethics and Moral Education*. Berkeley: University of California Press.

Nordam, A., K. Torjuul, V. Sorlie. 2005. Ethical challenges in the care of older people and risk of being burned out among male nurses. *Journal of Clinical Nursing* 14: 1248-56.

Nussbaum, Martha. 1992. *Love's Knowledge*. New York: Oxford University Press.

Nussbaum, Martha. 2000. *Women and Human Development: The Capabilities Approach*. New York: Cambridge University Press.

Nussbaum, Martha. 2001. *Upheavals of Thought. The Intelligence of Emotions*. Cambridge: University Press (especially 200-6; 342-50).

Nussbaum, Martha. 2002. Long-term care and social justice: A challenge to conventional ideas of the social contract. In *Ethical Choices in Long-Term Care: What does Justice Require?*, World Health Organization. Geneva: World Health Organization.

Nussbaum, Martha. 2004. *Hiding from Humanity: Disgust, Shame and the Law*. Princeton: University Press.

Nussbaum, Martha. 2006. *Frontiers of Justice: Disability, Nationality, Species Membership*. Cambridge, Mass.: The Belknap Press of Harvard University Press.

Oderwald, A. K. 1994. *Lijden tussen de regels*. Zoetermeer: Nationale Commissie Chronisch Zieken.

Oliver, Kelly. 2001. *Witnessing: Beyond Recognition*. Minneapolis: University of Minnesota Press.

*Oxford Advanced Learner's Dictionary of Current English*. 2005. Oxford: Oxford University Press.

Paley, John. 2002. Virtues of autonomy: The Kantian ethics of care. *Nursing Philosophy* 3: 133-43.

Parker, Pat. 2000. "FOR THE WHITE PERSON WHO WANTS TO KNOW HOW TO BE MY FRIEND " *Callaloo* 23 (1): 73.

Parreñas, Rhacel Salazar. 2001. *Servants of Globalization: Women, Migration, and Domestic Work*. Stanford, CA: Stanford University Press.

Plumwood, Val. 1993. *Feminism and the Mastery of Nature*. New York: Routledge.

Puchalski, Cristine M. 2002. Spirituality and end-of-life care: A time for listening and caring. *Journal of Palliative Medicine* 5: 289-94.

Rashotte, J. 2005. Dwelling with stories that haunt us: Building a meaningful nursing practice. *Nursing Inquiry* 12: 34-42.

Reader, Soran. 2007. The other side of agency. *Philosophy* 82: 579-604.

Reich, Warren. 2000. 'Sorge' in Goethes Faust. Goethe als Moralist. In *Erzählen und Moral: Narrativität im Spannungsfeld von Ethik und Äesthetik*, ed. D. Mieth, 143-65. Tübingen: Attempto.

Reich, Warren. 2004. History of the Notion of Care. In *Encyclopedia of Bioethics*, ed. S. Post, 349-61. New York: Thomson & Gale.

Ricoeur, Paul. 1990. *Soi-même comme un autre*. Paris: Seuil.

Ricoeur, Paul. 1992. *Oneself as Another*. London, Chicago: University of Chicago Press.

Roach, S. 1993. *The Human Act of Caring. A Blueprint for the Health Professions*. Ottawa: Canadian Hospital Association Press.

Rogers, Carl. 1963. A theory of therapy, personality and interpersonal relationships, as developed in the client-centered framework. In *Psychology: A Study of Science* vol. 3, ed. S. Koch, 184-256. New York: McGraw Hill.

Rousseau, Jean-Jacques. 1996. *Œuvres complètes*, III, Paris: Gallimard.

Rubenstein, Caren. 1993. Consumer's world: Finding a nanny legally. *The New York Times*, January 28, C 1.

Sabatino, C.J. 1999. Reflections on the meaning of care. *Nursing Ethics* 5: 383-9.

Schalock, R. et al. 2010. *Intellectual Disability: Definition, Classification, and Systems of Supports*. Washington: AAIDD.

Schechtman, Marya. 1996.*The Constitution of Selves*. New York: Cornell University Press.

Schnabl, Christa. 2004. Fürsorge zwischen kirchlichen Traditionen und feministischer Kritik. In *Ethik im Konflikt der Überzeugungen*, ed. Andreas Lob-Hüdepohl [Studien zur theologischen Ethik 105, Freiburg]

Schnabl, Christa. 2005. *Gerecht Sorgen: Grundlagen einer Sozialethischen Theorie der Fürsorge*. Fribourg/Wien.

Schnabl, Christa. 2008. Fürsorge. Eine Kategorie feministischer Ethik und ihre Bedeutung für die christliche Sozialethik. In *Feministische Ethik und christliche Sozialethik*, ed. Christian Spieß, Katja Winkler, 219-52. Berlin: Lit. [Schriften des Instituts für christliche Sozialwissenschaften der Westfälischen Wilhelms-Universität Münster Vol. 57]

Scully, Jackie Leach. 2009. Moral bodies: Epistemologies of embodiment. In *Naturalized Bioethics: Responsible Knowing and Practice*, ed. Marian Verkerk, Hilde Lindemann, and Margaret Urban Walker, 23-41. New York: Cambridge University Press.

Sen, Amartya. 1999. *Development as Freedom*. New York: Anchor Books.

Sennett, Richard. 2003. *Respect. The Formation of Character in an Age of Inequality*. New York.

Sevenhuijsen, Selma. 1998. *Citizenship and the Ethics of Care: Feminist Considerations on Justice, Morality and Politics*. New York: Routledge.

Sexton, J. B., E. J. Thomas, R. L. Helmreich. 2000. Error, stress and teamwork in medicine and aviation: Cross sectional surveys. *British Medical Journal* 320: 745-9.

Shapiro, J. 2008. Walking a mile in their patients' shoes: empathy and othering in medical students' education. *Philosophy, Ethics and Humanities* 3: 10.

Shortridge-Baggett, L. M. 2002. Self-efficacy: Measurement and intervention in nursing. In *Self-Efficacy in Nursing: Research and Measurement Perspectives*, ed. E.R. Lenz & L. M. Shortridge-Baggett. New York: Springer Publishing Company.

Silk, J. 1998. Caring at a distance. *Ethics, Place and Environment* 1: 165-82.

Simmes, F. & M. Grypdonck. 1999. Leven met type 2 diabetes. Een onderzoek onder mensen uit de lage sociaal-economische klasse. *TVZ. Tijdschrift voor Verpleegkundigen* 109: 648-52.

Singer, Peter. 2007. A convenient truth. *New York Times*. 26 Jan.

Smeyers, P. 1999. 'Care' and wider ethical issues. *Journal of Philosophy of Education* 33: 233-51.

Sölle, Dorothee. 1978. *Sympathie. Theologisch-politische Traktate*. Stuttgart: Kreuz Verlag.

Stepien K. A. & Baernstein A. 2006. Educating for empathy. A review. *Journal of General Internal Medicine* 21: 524-30.

Stocker, M. 1987. The schizophrenia of modern ethical theories. In *The Virtues: Contemporary Essays on Moral Character*, ed. R. B. Kruschwitz and R. C. Roberts. Belmont, CA: Wadsworth.

Sulmasy, Daniel P. 2006. Spiritual issues in the care of dying patients: "... It's okay between me and God." *Journal of the American Medical Association* 296: 1385-92.

Swanson, Jacinda. 2005. Recognition and Redistribution: Rethinking Culture and the Economic. *Theory, Culture & Society* 22: 87-118.

Taylor, Charles. 1994. The politics of recognition. In *Multiculturalism: Examining the Politics of Recognition*, ed. A. Gutmann, 25-73. Princeton: Princeton University Press.

Testerman J. K. et al. 1996. The natural history of cynicism in physicians. *Academic Medicine* 71: (supplement) s43-45.

Thomas Aquinas. *Summa Theologiae*. Latin text and English translation. Ed. Thomas Gilby, T. C. O'Brien (Blackfriars) 60 Vols, London-New York 1963-81.

Titchen, Angie. 2000. *Professional Craft Knowledge in Patient-centred Nursing and Facilitation of its Development*. Doctoral Dissertation. University of Oxford, UK.

Todorov, Tzvetan. 1995. *La vie commune. Essai d'anthropologie générale*. Paris: Seuil.

Tronto, Joan C. 1987. Beyond gender differences to a theory of care. *Signs* 12 (4): 644-62.

Tronto, Joan C. 1993. *Moral Boundaries: A Political Argument for an Ethic of Care*. New York: Routledge.

van der Laan, Geert. 2003. De professionele expert in practice-based evidence. *Sociale Interventie* 12 (4): 5-16.

van der Lans, Jos, Nies Medema, Marc Räkers. 2003. *Bemoeien werkt: naar een pragmatisch paternalisme in de sociale sector*. Amsterdam: De Balie.

van Gennep, A. 2000. *Emancipatie van de zwaksten in de samenleving. Over paradigma's van verstandelijke handicap*. Amsterdam: Boom.

van Heijst, Annelies. 2001. Zorgen, conventie, keuze of wat anders? (Seventeenth Socrates Lecture) *Tijdschrift voor Humanistiek* 6: 70-84.

van Heijst, Annelies. 2002. *Liefdewerk. Een herwaardering van de caritas bij de Arme Zusters van het Goddelijk Kind, sinds 1852*. Hilversum: Verloren.

van Heijst, Annelies. 2005. *Menslievende zorg. Een ethische kijk op professionaliteit*. Kampen: Klement.

van Heijst, Annelies. 2006a. Dignity as a relational concept: Arguments pro and contra from the ethics of care. In *Bodiliness and Human Dignity*, ed. Harm Goris, 89-97. Tilburg: Tilburg Theological Studies 2.

van Heijst, Annelies. 2006b. Menslievendheid: de essentie van zorg vanuit zorgethisch perspectief. In *Minder hard—meer hart! Zorgethiek en management: een werkzame combinatie*, ed. Annelies van Heijst, Thijs Tromp, Andries Baart, 9-20. Utrecht: Stichting Reliëf.

van Heijst, Annelies. 2008a. *Iemand zien staan. Zorgethiek over erkenning*. Kampen: Klement.

van Heijst, Annelies. 2008b. Zorgethiek, een theoretisch overzicht. *Filosofie en praktijk* 29 (1): 7-18.

van Heijst, Annelies. 2008c. Models of charitable care: catholic nuns and children in their care in Amsterdam, 1852-2002. Leiden: Brill (revision and translation of van Heijst 2002).

Vanlaere, Linus. 2006. *Zorg. Een wijsgerig- en theologisch-ethisch grondslagenonderzoek met de toepassing op de zorg voor suïcidale ouderen*. Leuven: PhD dissertation.

Vanlaere, Linus & Chris Gastmans. 2007. A normative approach to care ethics: The contribution of the Louvain tradition of personalism. In *New Pathways for Bioethics*, ed. Chris Gastmans, Kris Dierickx, Herman Nys and Paul Schotsmans. Antwerp & Oxford: Intersentia.

van Hooft, S. 1995. *Caring: An Essay in the Philosophy of Ethics*. Niwot, CO: University Press of Colorado.

van Tongeren, Paul. 1999. Activiteit en passiviteit. *Tijdschrift voor Gezondheidszorg en Ethiek* 9: 13-6.

Vehmas, S. 2004. Ethical analysis of the concept of disability. *Mental Retardation* 42 (3): 209-22.

Verhoeven, C. 2002. Belangeloze zorg. In *Op verhaal komen: Zorg en vragen naar zin*, ed. C. Vergeer. Eindhoven: Damon.

Verkerk, Marian ed. 1997. *Denken over zorg: Concepten en praktijken*, Utrecht.

Verkerk, Marian. 1999. A care perspective on coercion and autonomy. *Bioethics* 13 (3-4): 358-68.

Verkerk, Marian. 2007. Care ethics as a feminist perspective on bioethics. In *New Pathways for Bioethics*, ed. Chris Gastmans, Kris Dierickx, Herman Nys and Paul Schotsmans. Antwerp & Oxford: Intersentia 65-81.

Verkerk, Marian. 2005. A feminist care-ethics approach to genetics. In *Case Analysis in Clinical Ethics*, ed. R. Ashcroft, A. Lucassen, M. Parker, M. A. Verkerk and G. A. M. Widdershoven. Cambridge, Cambridge University Press: 133-49.

Vine, I. 1992. Altruism and human nature: Resolving the evolutionary paradox. In *Embracing the Other. Philosophical, Psychological, and Historical Perspectives on Altruism*, ed. P. M. Oliner, S. P. Oliner, L. Baron, L. A. Blum, D. L. Krebs, M. Z. Smolenska, 73-103. New York: University Press.

Vorstenbosch, Jan. 2005. *Zorg: Een filosofische analyse*. Amsterdam: Nieuwezijds.

Vosman, Frans. 1997. *De orde van het geluk: inleiding in de algemene moraaltheologie*. Baarn: Gooi en Sticht.

Vosman, Frans. 2001. *Goed gebleken: een doordenking van onzekerheid in traditionele moraaltheologische traktaten over onderscheidingsvermogen en scrupulositeit tegen de achtergrond van de hedendaagse tegenstelling objectieve en subjectieve moraal*. Utrecht: KTU 2001 (inaugural addres Katholieke Theologische Universiteit, Utrecht).

Vosman, Frans and Andries Baart. 2008. *Aannemelijke zorg. Over het uitzieden en verdringen van praktische wijsheid in de gezondheidszorg*. Den Haag: Lemma (joint inaugural address University of Tilburg).

Waerness, K. 1987. The rationality of caring. In *Women and the State*, ed. A. S. Sassoon. London: Hutchinson.

Walker, Margaret Urban. 2003. Human Conditions. In *Moral Contexts*, ed. Margaret Urban Walker. Lanham, Md.: Rowman & Littlefield.

Walker, Margaret Urban. 1998. *Moral Understandings*. New York: Routledge.

Walker, Margaret Urban. 2006. *Moral Repair: Reconstructing Moral Relations after Wrongdoing*. New York: Cambridge University Press.

Waterschoot, M. 2006. *Toetsen van een richtlijn ter bevordering van zelfmanagement van vochtbeperking*. Masterscriptie Verpleegkunde en Vroedkunde, Universiteit Gent.

Watson, J. 1985. *Nursing: Human Science and Human Care—A Theory of Nursing*. New York: National League for Nursing.

Watson, J. 2003. Love and caring: Ethics of face and hand. An invitation to return to the heart and soul of nursing and our deep humanity. *Nursing Administration Quarterly* 27: 197-202.

Waerness, Kari. 1990. Informal and formal care in old age: What is wrong with the new ideology in Scandinavia today? In *Gender and Caring: Work and Welfare in Britain and Scandinavia*, ed. C. Ungerson, 207-34. London: Harvester, Wheatsheaf.

Weggeman, M. 2000. *Kennismanagement: de praktijk*. Schiedam: Scriptum.

Weggeman, M. 2007. *Leidinggeven aan professionals? Niet doen! Over kenniswerkers, vakmanschap en innovatie*. Schiedam: Scriptum.

Weldam, S., M. J. Litjens, & M. Grypdonck. 2004. *Richtlijnontwikkeling voor bevordering van adequaat zelfmanagement met betrekking tot de vochtbeperking bij hemodialysepatiënten: een belevingsgerichte aanpak*. Disciplinegroep Verplegingswetenschap, Universiteit Utrecht.

Wendel, Saskia. 2003. *Feministische Ethik: Zur Einführung*. Hamburg.

Wendell, Susan. 1996. *The Rejected Body: Feminist Philosophical Reflections on Disability*. New York: Routledge.

*Werken aan balans: remedies tegen burn-out*. 2002. Den Haag: Raad voor Maatschappelijke Ontwikkeling/Den Haag: Sdu Uitgevers (Advice 22).

*Wikipedia. The Free Encyclopedia*. 2007. http://en.wikipedia.org

Willett, Cynthia. 2001. *The Soul of Justice: Social Bonds and Racial Hubris*, New York: Cornell University Press.

Williams, B. 1981. Persons, character, and morality. In *Moral Luck*. Cambridge University Press, New York.

Williams, G. 1993. Chronic illness and the pursuit of virtue in everyday life. In *Worlds of Illness: Biographical and Cultural Perspectives on Health and Disease*, ed. Alan Radley. London: Routledge.

Wilson, John R. S. 1977. In one another's power. *Ethics* 88: 299-315.

Young, I. M. 1997. Asymmetrical reciprocity: On moral respect, wonder, and enlarged thought. *Constellations* 3: 340-63.

# CONTRIBUTORS

**Andries Baart** is a Professor of Presence and Care at Tilburg University. He is the founder of the so-called theory of presence and the (practice orientated) presence-approach. He is also the impelling force behind the Presence Foundation, a platform for research and practice innovation in professional health care and welfare. Some of his key publications are: *Een theorie van de presentie* (2001) [A Theory of Presence]; together with Frans Vosman *Present* (2003) [Present]; *Aandacht* (2005) [Attentiveness]; *Kwetsbaar maar niet alleen kwetsbaar* (2007) [Vulnerable, but more than just vulnerable]; together with Mieke Grypdonck *Verpleegkunde en presentie* (2008) [Nursing and Presence]; and together with Frans Vosman *Aannemelijke zorg* (2008) [Plausible Care].

**Estelle Ferrarese** is an Assistant Professor of Political Theory at the University of Strasbourg and a researcher at Laboratoire Cultures et Société en Europe. Her central research topics are the struggle for recognition, feminist political theory, deliberative democracies, German political philosophy, and the relation between recognition and vulnerability. She has published several works and reviews and is the co-editor, with Nancy Fraser, of *Qu'est-ce que la justice sociale? Reconnaissance et redistribution* (2005).

**Chris Gastmans** obtained his PhD in theology in 1995. He is a Professor of Medical Ethics at the Centre for Biomedical Ethics and Law of the Faculty of Medicine, Catholic University of Leuven, Belgium. He is also Secretary-General of the European Association of Centres of Medical Ethics (EACME). His most important publications are *Between Technology and Humanity* (2002) and *New Pathways for European Bioethics* (2007). He published articles in international journals and books on nursing ethics, ethics of care, end-of-life care and elderly care.

**Mieke Grypdonck** is a Professor in Nursing Theory who worked at the Universities of Leuven, Utrecht, and Ghent. She is interested in methods and theories that further a more humane type of professional nursing care. She developed a model of nursing care for patients with a chronic illness. Mieke Grypdonck uses both qualitative and quantitative research. She introduced the approach of integrative nursing, with special attention for the wholeness of human individuals. In 2009, she has been given emeritus status.

**Emmanuel Housset** is a Lecturer at the Department of Philosophy of the University of Caen-Low-Normandy (UCBN) and member of his team of Identity research and subjectivity. Specialist in phenomenology, he wrote two books on Husserl and a study of the phenomenology of passions: *L'intelligence de la pitié. Phénoménologie de la communauté* (2003) [The Intelligence of Pity. Phenomenology of Communality]. Recently he wrote two books on personal identity: *La vocation de la personne* (2007) [The Personal Calling] and *L'intériorité d'exil* (2008) [The Interiority in Exile].

**Carlo Leget** is an Associate Professor of the Ethics of Care at Tilburg University. He has a PhD in theology (1997) from the Catholic Theological University at Utrecht, where he taught moral theology until 2002. He worked from 2002-2008 as Associate Professor of Medical Ethics at the Radboud University Nijmegen Medical Centre. The Ethics of Care and spirituality are his main areas of professional activity. He has specialized in subjects such as palliative care, the ethics of end-of-life questions, the art of living and dying, and the place of spirituality in palliative care. He authored *Living with God. Thomas Aquinas on the Relation between Life on Earth and 'Life' after Death* (1997), *Ruimte om te sterven* (2003) [A Space to Die] and *Van levenskunst tot stervenskunst* (2008) [From the art of living to the art of dying].

**Axel Liégeois** is Professor of Practical Theology at the Faculty of Theology of the Catholic University of Leuven, and ethical advisor at the Brothers of Charity in Gent, Belgium. His field of research is care ethics and pastoral care, especially for people with psychiatric problems or with intellectual disability. He published several articles and the following books: *Begrensde vrijheid. Ethiek in de geestelijke gezondheidszorg* [Limited Freedom] (1997); *Geestkracht. Pastoraat en geestelijke gezondheidszorg* [Spiritual Strength] (2004); *Schroomvol nabij. Pastorale begeleiding bij euthanasie* [Respectful Presence] (2008); *Waarden in dialoog. Ethiek in de zorg* [Values in Dialogue] (2009).

**Hilde Lindemann** is Professor of Philosophy at Michigan State University. A Fellow of the Hastings Center and past president of the American Society for Bioethics and Humanities, she is a former editor of *Hypatia*. Her books include *Damaged Identities, Narrative Repair* (2001), *An Invitation to Feminist Ethics* (2005), and the recently coedited *Naturalized Bioethics: Toward Responsible Knowing and Practice* (2008). Her ongoing research interests are in narrative approaches to bioethics, feminist ethics, the ethics of families, and the social construction of persons and their identities.

**Christa Schnabl** is Associate Professor at the Institute for Social Ethics at the Catholic Faculty of Theology in Vienna. She is also appointed as vice-president of the University of Vienna. She did research on welfare service and politics. She is author of the book *Das Moralische im Politischen. Zur Normativität des Handelns bei Hannah Arendt im Kontext der theologischen Ethik* (1999) [The Moral dimension of Politics] and *Gerecht sorgen. Grundlagen einer sozialethischen Theorie der Fürsorge* (2005) [Justified Care]. Main research fields are political theory, justice and care, ethics in the dialogue with Hannah Arendt, ethics and gender, welfare service, ethics of care and politics.

**Joan Tronto** is Professor of Political Science at the University of Minnesota. She has held visiting appointments at Yale University, the University of Humanist Studies, the Netherlands, the University of Bologna, and at Goethe University in Frankfurt-am-Main. Tronto has authored numerous articles and *Moral Boundaries: A Political Argument for an Ethic of Care* (1993). She is the co-editor, with Cathy Cohen and Kathy Jones, of *Women Transforming Politics: An Alternative Reader* (1997). Tronto received Hunter College's Faculty Award for Teaching Excellence in 1991. Her co-authored (with Stephen Leonard) 2007 essay, "The Genders of Citizenship," co-won the first annual Okin-Young Award for feminist political theory awarded by the American Political Science Association.

**Annelies van Heijst** is professor of Care, Culture and Charity at the Tilburg University. Her academic research hinges around the actual and historical connections between 'love' and 'care'. The research has two focus points. The first is on professional care in its current cultural context—resulting in various articles and two books *Menslievende zorg* [Professional loving care] published in 2005, and *Iemand zien staan* [Recognizing the other] released in 2008. The second research focus point is on the history of charity, as carried out in the nineteenth and twentieth centuries by Catholic nuns in the public sphere. This resulted in *Liefdewerk. Een herwaardering van de caritas van de Arme Zusters van het Goddelijk Kind sinds 1852*, which was published in 2002. An enlarged English edition appeared in 2008 as *Models of charitable Care. Catholic Nuns and Children in their Care in Amsterdam, 1852-2002.* Together with the historians Marjet Derks and Marit Monteiro she co-authored an historical overview of two centuries of Dutch charity, entitled *Ex Caritate* (2010).

**Linus Vanlaere** obtained his PhD in theology in 2006, studying the ethical and philosophical foundations of care ethics. This research also contains an analysis, based on care ethics, of the clinical issues surrounding suicide among older persons. The project was funded by the National Fund for Scientific Research Flanders (FWO) and was realised at the Centre for Biomedical Ethics and Law under supervision of Prof. Dr. Chris Gastmans. Vanlaere is currently working as a clinical ethicist in a group of eight nursing homes in Flanders, Belgium. He is also scientific researcher in sTimul: care-ethics lab (Moorsele, Belgium). sTimul is a surprising and innovative way of stimulating care ethics in elderly care.

**Frans Vosman** is professor of Christian Ethics and Spirituality at the Tilburg University. He focuses on politico-ethical and socio-ethical questions and on the politico-ethical reflection of issues that are often regarded as an individual-ethical, private matter (e.g. sex, the ending of human life.) In this he lets himself be guided by the rich and very relevant catholic moral traditions. Frans Vosman published several articles. He resorts to, amongst others, the theories of Charles Larmore, Michael Walzer, and Paul Ricoeur (philosophical ethics). He also takes a keen interest in contemporary French phenomenology. Research topics: bioethics, elderly people, ethics, intercultural ethics, intercultural theology, medical ethics, moral theology, occupational ethics, political philosophy/political ethics.

**Margaret Urban Walker** is Professor of Philosophy and Lincoln Professor of Ethics at the Philosophy Faculty, School of Historical, Philosophical, and Religious Studies, Arizona State University. Her areas of specialization are Anglo-American ethics and political theory, reparative and restorative justice, moral psychology, feminist ethics, and Wittgenstein. She is author of *Moral Understandings: A Feminist Study in Ethics*, 2nd Edition (2007); *Moral Contexts* (2003); *Moral Repair: Reconstructing Moral Relations after Wrongdoing* (2006); and *What is Reparative Justice?* (2010). She is editor or co-editor of *Mother Time: Women, Aging, and Ethics* (1998); *Moral Psychology*, with Peggy DesAutels (2004); and *Naturalized Bioethics*, with Hilde Lindemann and Marian Verkerk (2009). Her current work focuses on issues of reparation, truth-telling, forgiveness, and justice in the aftermath of serious wrongs.

INDEX

PRINTED ON PERMANENT PAPER • IMPRIME SUR PAPIER PERMANENT • GEDRUKT OP DUURZAAM PAPIER - ISO 9706

N.V. PEETERS S.A., WAROTSTRAAT 50, B-3020 HERENT